ROGER J. BULGER
MARIAN OSTERWEIS
ELAINE R. RUBIN
EDITORS

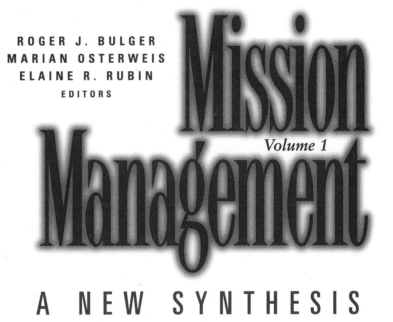

Mission Management

Volume 1

A NEW SYNTHESIS

ASSOCIATION OF ACADEMIC HEALTH CENTERS

The Association of Academic Health Centers (AHC) is a national, nonprofit organization representing more than 100 institutional members in the United States that are the health complexes of the major universities. Academic health centers consist of an allopathic or osteopathic school of medicine, at least one other health professions school or program, and one or more teaching hospitals. These institutions are the nation's primary resources for education in the health professions, biomedical and health services research, and many aspects of patient care.

The AHC seeks to influence public dialogue on significant health and science policy issues, to advance education for health professionals, to promote biomedical and health services research, and to enhance patient care. The AHC is dedicated to improving the health of the people through leadership and cooperative action with others.

Library of Congress Cataloging-in-Publication Data

Mission management: a new synthesis / Roger J. Bulger, Marian Osterweis, Elaine R. Rubin, editors.

     p.   cm.

   Includes bibliographical references (p.).

   ISBN 1-879694-13-1 (v. 1)

   1. Academic medical centers- -United States.   I. Bulger, Roger J.

RA981. A2M56 1998

362.1' 0973—dc21   98-19149

                                                    CIP

Available from:
Association of Academic Health Centers
1400 Sixteenth Street, N.W., Suite 720
Washington, D. C. 20036
202/265-9600; Fax 202/265-7514
Price: $25.00 (plus $5.00 shipping/handling)

Design and production by Fletcher Design, Washington, DC

Copy editing by SSR, Inc.

CONTENTS

Association of Academic Health Centers
STUDY COMMITTEE

Roger J. Bulger, M.D.
President
Association of Academic Health Centers
Chair

Robert J. Baker, M.B.A.
President and Chief Executive Officer
University HealthSystem Consortium

Dennis C. Brimhall
President
University of Colorado Hospital
 Authority

Gerard N. Burrow, M.D.
Special Advisor to the President for
 Health Affairs and
David Paige Smith Professor of Medicine
Yale University

Mary Sue Coleman, Ph.D.
President
The University of Iowa

Michael J. Halseth
Executive Director, University of Virginia
 Medical Center
University of Virginia

Donald C. Harrison, M.D.
Senior Vice President and Provost for
 Health Affairs
University of Cincinnati Medical Center

Leo M. Henikoff, M.D.
President and Chief Executive Officer
Rush-Presbyterian-St. Luke's Medical
 Center

Thomas H. Jackson, J.D.
President and Chief Executive Officer
University of Rochester

Peter O. Kohler, M.D.
President
Oregon Health Sciences University

Aaron Lazare, M.D.
Chancellor and Dean of the School of
 Medicine
University of Massachusetts Medical
 Center

Russell Miller, M.D.
President Emeritus
State University of New York Health
 Science Center at Brooklyn

Ralph W. Muller
President
University of Chicago Hospitals and
 Health Systems

William Petasnick
President and Chief Executive Officer
Froedtert Memorial Lutheran
 Hospital, Inc.

Ralph Snyderman, M.D.
Chancellor for Health Affairs
Dean, School of Medicine and
 President and Chief Executive Officer
Duke University Health System
Duke University Medical Center

Graham B. Spanier, Ph.D.
President
The Pennsylvania State University

Consultant:
Kaludis Consulting Group

CONTRIBUTORS

Sage Bennet, PhD, is associate professor of health professions, Western University of Health Sciences.

Julien F. Biebuyck, MB, DPhil, is senior associate dean for academic affairs, College of Medicine, The Pennsylvania State University.

T. Michael Bolger, JD, is president and chief executive officer, The Medical College of Wisconsin.

Roger J. Bulger, MD, is president, Association of Academic Health Centers.

Patricia Chase, PhD, is professor of pharmacy practice and facilitative officer for the Division of Professional Education, Western University of Health Sciences.

Lois Davis is director of corporate communications, Oregon Health Sciences University.

C. McCollister Evarts, MD, is senior vice president for health affairs, The Pennsylvania State University; dean, College of Medicine, The Pennsylvania State University; and president and chief academic officer, Penn State Geisinger Health System.

R.K. Dieter Haussmann, PhD, is vice chancellor for health services, University of Illinois at Chicago.

Leo M. Henikoff, MD, is president and chief executive officer, Rush-Presbyterian-St. Luke's Medical Center.

Richard Janeway, MD, is former executive vice president for health affairs at Wake Forest University and chief executive officer, Bowman Gray School of Medicine.

The Kaludis Consulting Group is a Washington, DC-based firm specializing in consultation on higher education and academic health centers.

Peter O. Kohler, MD, is president, Oregon Health Sciences University.

Craig S. Kuehn, PhD, is associate professor of anatomy, Western University of Health Sciences.

John C. LaRosa, MD, is chancellor, Tulane University Medical Center.

Jonathan Leo, PhD, is assistant professor of anatomy, Western University of Health Sciences.

Robert Michels, MD, is former provost/medical affairs, Cornell University, and dean, Cornell University Medical Center.

Reverend Michael G. Morrison, SJ, is president, Creighton University.

Richard O'Brien, MD, is vice president for health sciences, Creighton University.

Marian Osterweis, PhD, is executive vice president, Association of Academic Health Centers.

Harry Rosenberg, PharmD, PhD, is professor of pharmaceutical sciences and dean (chief facilitative officer), Western University of Health Sciences.

Elaine R. Rubin, PhD, is assistant vice president for program, Association of Academic Health Centers.

Carl E. Trinca, PhD, is professor of pharmacy education, vice provost/vice president for strategic planning, Western University of Health Sciences.

Kern Wildenthal, MD, PhD, is president, The University of Texas Southwestern Medical Center at Dallas.

Rafi Younoszai, PhD, is professor of anatomy, Western University of Health Sciences.

PREFACE

THE FUTURE OF SCIENTIFICALLY GROUNDED HEALTH care has never been more promising. The genetics revolution is in its infancy, but already the spectacular fruits of molecular biological research are starting to make their appearance in clinical practice. The advance of information sciences, including computerization and the Internet, promises to have profound effects on the health care sector. Indeed, combined with advances in the clinical evaluative sciences, patient outcome measurement and disease management techniques, information sciences offer the possibility of implementing health care delivery systems with far greater effectiveness, far greater efficiency, and far more accessibility than ever before.

These revolutionary events provide unprecedented opportunities for academic health centers to integrate their missions in ways never before possible. Today's scientific advances, however, also coincide with a period of unprecedented changes in the financing and organization of health care services. Although science is dramatically expanding the horizons for health care delivery, many people fear that managed care and overriding concerns about the costs of health care may compromise future scientific inquiry, the translation of scientific breakthroughs to bedside care, and the education of future health professionals.

In 1997, therefore, the Association of Academic Health Centers undertook a study of the impact of and challenges posed by dramatic changes in financing and delivery of health care services on academic health centers, particularly on their academic mission (that is, education and research).

Public demands and expectations related to cost, efficiency, and accountability that have reverberated through corporate America are now affecting higher education, and compounding the economic and marketplace challenges already facing universities and academic health centers. Institutional and professional questions about the nature of health professions education and advances in science and technology are heightening pressures to change the status quo and are quickening the pace of change.

Until recently, the organization and structure of academic health centers has been little studied. In addition, little attention has been paid to the education and research missions of academic health centers as these institutions restructure in response to changes affecting health care services. Of great concern is that the capacity of academic health centers to provide education and research has not only been threatened by shrinking funds but also overshadowed by an enormous preoccupation with the financing and organization of clinical services.

In contrast, the service enterprise of the academic health center has been well studied. Most institutions have developed strategies for dealing with their local environments, which often involve freeing the clinical service enterprise of the academic health center from university or state bureaucracies and creating integrated, flexible operations, capable of developing and implementing contracts, relationships, and strategies necessary for the survival of the university's teaching hospitals and associated patient activities.

This AHC study not only examines significant organizational issues but also takes account of new external forces that are transforming the two unique but interconnected worlds of higher education and health care delivery. We see academic health centers and universities in a period of uncertainty, with issues of competition and entrepreneurial activities threatening to unseat traditional missions and to create financial crises. But we also see these institutions responding to new environments and adapting for the future.

As a variety of forces emerge to unbalance the traditional education, research, and service missions, so too have institutional strategies and initiatives developed to create a new synthesis between the mission components. From new structures and management systems to different educational philosophies and research organizations, leaders of academic health centers are helping to transform these institutions to ensure survival and balance of the mission components. These times, however daunting, are providing opportunities for leaders of academic health centers to reshape the institutional mission and to find innovative ways to ensure that the unique and valuable institutional functions that academic health centers have provided to society are protected and maintained.

Finally, this study offers insights into the strategies and innovations these institutions are employing to meet their complex challenges. In so doing, the study provides information for understanding the growth, evolution, and survival of institutions while opening a window on societal change. From changing Federal and state funding to the growth of managed care, and from public demands for increased accountability and responsiveness to community needs to the impact of scientific and technological advances, the study provides a snapshot of the impact of political and socioeconomic forces on academic health centers—institutions whose work has been synonymous with societal interests in the realms of health education, research, and service.

As we look back on the 1990s, we may find that this decade marked a turning point for universities and academic health centers in relations with their communities. The traditional commitment to the community on the part of these institutions, fostered in part by a heightened sense of accountability and service, is being renewed and expanded.

Academic health centers, in particular, are redefining their service mission and emerging to take leading roles in myriad activities from health promotion to economic development in inner cities. Academic health centers are redirecting their expertise in research and education to increasingly serve their communities beyond the realm of patient care. Whether conducting science classes at local high schools, sponsoring Head Start programs, or renovating inner city housing, the academic health center commitment to community service is finding expression.

This book, volume 1 in a two-volume study entitled *Mission Management: A New Synthesis*, is the final report of the Study Committee.

The study sought to accomplish the following tasks.

1. Understand the influence of health care and economic forces and examine their impact on the academic health center's education and research missions.

2. Examine issues of organization, governance, leadership, and financing as they relate to each mission individually and to the academic health center–university relationship as a whole.

3. Identify a range of models and strategies characteristic of successful

academic health centers in today's environment, including relationships among their own components and with their parent universities and communities.

Multiple, mostly qualitative, methods were employed to analyze the issues, understand institutional responses, and tease out the lessons to be learned from a variety of experiences and professional perspectives. These included the following:

- Commissioning a set of background papers from experts in higher education, institutional leadership, culture, health professions education, biomedical research, health services, organizational behavior, and the globalization of health. These have been published as volume 2.

- Querying all member-representatives of the Association of Academic Heath Centers about changes in structure, governance, financing, and organization, both overall and in relation to each of the mission areas at their institutions in order to get a broad sense of what is happening in this universe.

- Conducting in-depth site visits to four academic health centers to glean details about some institutions with interesting approaches to restructuring, designed to help them continue to accomplish their missions.

- Developing eleven case studies from presentations made at meetings of the Association of Academic Health Centers over the past two years, each one highlighting a particular aspect of the institutional mission and the strategies used to effect desired change.

Volume 1 begins with the observations, conclusions, and recommendations of the Study Committee, both in general and also specific to each of the three missions: education, research, and patient care. Chapter 1 is an overview of the eleven case studies. The survey results make up chapter 2; the site visit report is in chapter 3. A paper by Dr. Julien F. Biebuyck on the development of the new role of the clinical chair highlights one of the most significant elements of change and synthesis and appears in chapter 4.

The case studies themselves appear in appendix A. The majority of the case studies were written by Elaine R. Rubin, PhD, assistant vice president for program at the Association of Academic Health Centers, in collaboration with the AHC member who presented the case. We would again like to thank these members for sharing their institutional experiences: T. Michael Bolger, JD, president and chief executive officer, Medical College of Wisconsin; C. McCollister Evarts, MD, senior vice president for health affairs, dean, college of medicine and president and chief academic officer, Pennsylvania State Geisinger Health System; Leo M. Henikoff, MD, president and chief executive officer, Rush-Presbyterian-St. Luke's Medical Center; R. K. Dieter Haussmann, PhD, vice chancellor for health services, University of Illinois at Chicago; Richard Janeway, MD, former executive vice president for health affairs of Wake Forest University and chief executive officer, Bowman Gray School of Medicine; John C. LaRosa, MD, chancellor, Tulane University Medical Center; Robert Michels, MD, former provost/medical affairs and dean, Cornell University Medical Center; Richard L. O'Brien, MD, vice president for health sciences, Creighton University; Philip Pumerantz, PhD, president, and his colleagues, Western University of Health Sciences; Kern Wildenthal, MD, PhD, president, University of Texas Southwestern Medical Center at Dallas.

A committee, comprising university presidents, CEOs of academic health centers, university health system and hospital CEOs, and the president of the Association of Academic Health Centers, directed the study. The association's board of directors provided oversight for the entire project and also reviewed and approved the final report.

The study would not have been possible without the generous support of a number of organizations and the dedication of numerous individuals. We are grateful for the financial support provided by the Robert Wood Johnson Foundation, the University HealthSystem Consortium, and the Commonwealth Fund. We also appreciate the help and insights provided by the Kaludis Consulting Group, who conducted the site visits and shared with us the wisdom of their wide experience in education and academic health center management.

We hope that the study will be of use to administrators and faculty in academic health centers nationwide, to the higher education community, and to policymakers as they seek to make institutional changes that will ensure the appropriate attention to mission and values in the future.

RJB

MO

ERR

OBSERVATIONS, CONCLUSIONS, AND RECOMMENDATIONS

THE FOLLOWING SET OF OBSERVATIONS, CONCLU-
sions, and recommendations are set forth by the Study
Committee. We hope that they will be of use to academic health
centers, to the higher education community, and to policy-makers as they seek to make institutional changes that will ensure the appropriate
attention to mission and values in the future.

GENERAL OBSERVATIONS

*1. During this time of extraordinary change in health care, most academic health
centers are taking steps to alter their programs and structures in order to fulfill
their potential in the new age and to ensure financial solvency and long-term
survival.*

2. No single model is right for all academic health centers.

- Institutional history, culture, and mission, as well as local circumstances and characteristics of their parent universities and university
  systems (where these exist) will necessarily shape the strategies chosen
  by individual academic health centers. Some institutions are for the
  first time consolidating the health sciences under a vice president.
  Others, having separated the clinical function, have eliminated the vice
  president and assigned the integrative functions elsewhere, usually in
  the provost's or president's office; still others have split the health sciences off into a separate entity under the university president.

3. Change necessarily involves deep cultural shifts; it alters roles of leaders at all levels and has a tremendous impact on faculty and their traditions.

- "Transition management," as it has come to be called, is altering the roles of presidents, vice presidents, and deans. Perhaps the greatest stress is on the traditional job description of the departmental chairs. No longer, in many institutions, will they control all or most aspects of the research, education, and health services carried out in their departments. Integration and scale may drive them to being primarily recruiters and developers of talent, while exerting shared power through groups of leaders in each mission area.

4. As complexity and competition increase in this cost-conscious environment, strategy and focus are increasingly important factors for the success of academic health centers.

- Increasingly, these centers are moving toward "mission management" to achieve their goals and away from the traditional departmental or discipline-based approach.

5. Clinical restructuring provides an opportunity to consider organizational restructuring across the academic health center or the university that would align faculty to work in functional units while remaining within academic departments.

6. To ensure the integration of the academic (i.e., education and research) missions with the new clinical environment, leaders must develop and communicate a vision of institutional goals and priorities.

7. When major institutional change is decided upon, those institutions that can forge a strong shared vision among the top leaders (including at a minimum, the CEO of the academic health center, the university president, the provost where applicable, and the key leadership of the governing board) have the greatest likelihood of engineering creative change.

8. Societal forces, both governmental and market-generated, are raising to an unprecedented degree the emphasis on accountability for the institution as a whole and for individual faculty members.

9. Even as financing and societal realities push toward separating the management of the service, research, and education enterprises, other forces call for a new, yet different, level of reintegration across the academic enterprise.

GENERAL CONCLUSIONS AND RECOMMENDATIONS

1. Academic health centers should establish appropriate organizational venues to manage each of their mission areas (education, research, patient care, and community service).

- If these missions are managed separately, arrangements should be made to allow for the necessary integrative institutionwide effort. Ideally, institutionwide leadership and integration should be vested in one person or one office, whether that person is the vice president for health affairs, provost, or president.

2. As each organizational unit is put in place, the following matters must be addressed: ownership, governance, leadership, organization, and financing.

- For example, the institution must seek to develop an ever more sophisticated level of informed governance, which generally means that a core of influential trustees must understand the academic health center, be able to critique its efforts, and support what it is trying to do.

3. Executives must be risk-takers and must be allowed to make occasional mistakes, but also must earn trust through appropriate communication with all stakeholders.

4. Academic health centers must develop strategies that focus on targeted priorities and link them to resource allocation and reward systems.

- This process imperative is required to develop the infrastructure to facilitate new institutional (faculty and staff) behaviors.

5. Leadership and management are both required for success and must increasingly be firmly anchored in clearly stated values.

- This leadership imperative is required to implement the often-dramatic institutional reconfigurations necessary if institutional goals are to be realized. Succession planning and mentoring are critical elements to the continued development of excellent leaders and leadership capacity.

6. *The successful academic health center of the future must be oriented toward institutional goals and objectives and not based solely on individual disciplines, schools, or professions.*

7. *Cost concerns and an increasing constituency demand for accountability require that academic health centers develop and make known their performance metrics and benchmarks in all mission areas, including more sophisticated surrogate outcome measures in patient care and the health status of populations served.*

8. *Investment in information systems must be dramatically increased in most academic health centers.*

- As academic health centers move off campus to other institutional sites and even to individual offices and homes for education, research, patient care, and community service activities, the information infrastructure will become of premier importance in planning capital investments and tracking and coordinating activities in all spheres. Furthermore, appropriate and efficient information transfer is crucial to achieving the delicate balance between centralization of planning, resource allocation, and outcome evaluation, on the one hand, and decentralization with proper power and accountability of the management function on the other hand.

Education: Observations

1. *The higher education world is experiencing intense forces for change analogous to those that continue to buffet the health care industry. Fundamental societal concerns about cost, quality, and access in education have led to a rising crescendo of public opinion demanding accountability, evaluation, and a student/learning focus.*

2. *Education's importance has been devalued by the dominance of the patient care and research missions in many academic health centers.*

- Financial rewards and academic status come to the successful clinical specialist and to the topflight researcher, and seldom follow on excellence in the education arena.

3. Changes in the health care delivery system and the health care needs of an aging, increasingly diverse population are most effectively met when there is collaboration across the health professions and coordination with related social support services. Emphasis on interdisciplinary education remains low despite the shift of care to an interdisciplinary team approach.

- Most health professionals will be required to participate in interdisciplinary teams in order to better manage comprehensive care of patients and health plan enrollees. The current approach to health professions education provides little opportunity for students in the different professions to work together. Interdisciplinary clinical learning and practice experiences foster development of team skills, challenge stereotypes, and erode barriers between the professions.

- Current restructuring efforts are heavily concentrated on the clinical enterprise and the medical school. Yet any clinical partnership, merger, or separation is likely to affect clinical experiences for students in all the health professions, either directly or through the responses of competitors who provide teaching sites to other professions. There is too little attention paid to the clinical education needs of nursing, pharmacy, dentistry, and the allied health professions as mergers and partnerships are planned. Without sufficient attention, nonphysician health education programs could be adversely affected by a partnership.

4. The advances in information science have expanded dramatically the possibilities for both synchronous and asynchronous distance learning.

- Many exciting examples and models are being put in place and studied in health professions education.

5. Faculty performance reviews in health professions schools are becoming the rule rather than the exception. Although the complex job of accurately measuring faculty productivity in education, research, patient care, and administration is proving difficult, there are some successful models in place that offer the prospect of effectively linking faculty productivity with faculty income by area of faculty effort.

Education: Conclusions and Recommendations

1. Quality teaching must be valued and rewarded. This development requires major changes in faculty incentives and reward structures, including promotion and tenure, and significant attention to the development of proper benchmarks for education.

2. Students at all levels in all the health professions must be mentored in order to ensure that graduates are well prepared for and have realistic expectations about careers in education, research, and patient care.

3. Appropriate educational integration across disciplines, across specialties, and across professions must be encouraged and financially rewarded if patient care is to be delivered efficiently by a seamless web of interrelating and collaborating professionals.

4. Research in educational technique, outcomes, and innovation should become a major institutional emphasis.

- As curricula are often dramatically revised and new education techniques and technologies are introduced, evaluation of major new advances must be ongoing in order to ensure integration of quality teaching and technology in the educational environment.

5. Ongoing and consistent cost analyses of education must be widely adopted.

- Such quantitative data and analysis are essential for developing and implementing a plan and strategy for the education enterprise.

6. The analog of a "business" plan for education should be developed.

- Such a plan will identify goals, costs, income, and capital needs. It should allow for expenditures on innovation and develop a performance-based reward system with positive incentives to encourage faculty and staff productivity.

7. As resources decline and pressure for accountability rises, it may be in the interest of both academic health center and parent university to pursue new alliances in education and/or research.

- This effort might include considering whether basic science departments should assume responsibility for undergraduate teaching and/or creating research or policy institutes that cut across academic health centers and other university departments or divisions.

8. *Ownership/Governance.*

- The education effort is clearly within the purview of, and is "owned" and "governed" by the academic institution even though some clinical sites may not be so owned or governed. The clients or people to be served are the students.

9. *Leadership.*

- Planning, strategizing, integrating, implementing, and evaluating must all be done or coordinated centrally at the academic health center or university, although any particular step should be delegated to the site closest to where the education is occurring. The growing emphasis upon multiprofessional and interdisciplinary team education will require a supra- or trans-schools leadership venue.

10. *Finances for education must be managed such that return on investment can be shown in one convincing form or another.*

- Health professions schools in general, and medical schools in particular, can no longer afford to maintain that they cannot ascertain a figure for the cost of education because of their institutions' several funding streams and the three major joint products in education, in research, and in patient care. Cross-subsidies must be identified and agreed to prospectively. Cost-reducing techniques and steps must be sought and implemented, especially as fiscal support for education is diminishing in some places. Information must flow freely between practice sites and the central office so that integrative expenditure decisions can be made.

11. *Organization.*

- There is an obvious necessity to establish the appropriate level of integrative authority and accountability at the departmental, school, academic health center, and university levels. New forms of organization may be required to achieve the desired level of integration. At a very broad level, strong integrated advocacy is required, for example, to ensure that the institution's technology transfer apparatus is as open to, and as respectful of, educational technologic innovations as it is regarding research advances.

Research: Observations

1. Many observers worry that basic biomedical and clinical research is being increasingly concentrated in a smaller number of institutions. As "big science" increasingly requires large capital investments of financial and human resources, this trend will continue to highlight some thirty to forty institutions as research intensive. However, there are other important and exciting research opportunities for other institutions, most notably in the realms of health services and policy research and educational research.

2. Several major universities have moved significantly down the path toward establishing a coordinated approach to the management of the research enterprise.

- These efforts include sophisticated technology transfer activities leading to new and expanded income streams from faculty inventions and innovations. Attention is now turning increasingly to cost-control interventions, such as performance-based central space management and advanced information systems, which combine the benefits of large purchasing contracts with the decentralization of decision-making.

3. With the growing academic involvement with commerce and industry, there is evidence of increasing conflicts and compromises involving the traditional academic values of free communication of discovery and intellectual capital.

4. Biomedical research in the twenty-first century cannot usefully be delineated within or categorized by any single traditional departmental structure, such as anatomy or biochemistry or physiology.

Research: Conclusions and Recommendations

1. Every academic health center should have a research portfolio. And that portfolio should be consistent with its culture, its resources, and its missions.

- Some academic health centers and some health professions schools within them will emphasize basic biomedical and clinical research;

others will concentrate more on the applied and evaluative realms, such as health services research, epidemiologic studies, and assessment of new educational techniques.

2. The research enterprise at the academic health center should be managed in a business-like fashion.

- This recommendation suggests that a business plan be established for the entire enterprise that identifies what in business jargon would be the "product lines," but in this instance it would identify in the academic health center's own terms the separate activities to be managed within its research portfolio (e.g., basic laboratory research, clinical research, large-scale clinical trials, translational research aimed at product development, health services research, and clinical evaluative sciences).

- Research support services activities also need to be organized to better meet the goals of the entire enterprise. Thus, information systems, financial, space, and personnel management will also be accountable to their "customers" in light of a cost-conscious, mission-oriented effort. This approach will ensure that costs will be under constant review; waste and duplication will be under constant attack; capital investments will be carefully planned to meet both short- and long-term goals; and sources of financial support will be identified and managed according to an expenditure plan based upon the achievement of the mission.

- Each institution needs to set its objectives and establish benchmarks for achieving them, against which faculty researchers' productivity can be measured.

3. Coupled with appropriate attention to enhancing efficiency, care also must be taken to protect and preserve the traditional university environment that encourages faculty creativity in the discovery of new knowledge, and the dissemination of knowledge through teaching and publishing.

4. As a new research organization emerges, the committee recommends that careful attention be given to the following:

- Ownership of the research enterprise clearly must rest with the university. The administration and services run by the university must, however, be clear in their goals, that is, to serve the faculty and facilitate the efficient conduct of research by the investigators while meeting the compliance and regulatory standards of the government, the university, and the scientific community. The most proximal clients or people being served are the faculty researchers, although in the long run the public is the ultimate beneficiary of biomedical research.

- Governance must be inclusive of those being served by much of the enterprise (i.e., the researchers) and is best led by an individual who has the trust and respect of the research community.

- Leadership should rest in the hands of a research CEO whose job is to support the faculty in their efforts, to manage the mission, to develop and implement the business plan, and to continually tap outside and inside resources to help determine the critical investment choices for the various types of research. The leader must also be adept at shaping and reshaping the organization.

- Organization will no longer be defined solely in terms of departments and schools, although such units will not likely disappear or be unimportant. Rather, new entities will come into being such as mission-oriented centers and institutes, groupings around specific functions such as translational research, and the clinical evaluative sciences. With the emergence of such interdepartmental and cross-school centers, issues about who or what gets credit for research dollars brought in by their participants should be anticipated and planned for carefully.

- Financing must be based on accurate assessments of the costs of doing business, so that the magnitude of any institutional investment or cross-subsidy can be predetermined. This is essential to set development and fund-raising goals. Capital investment decisions should track the overall strategic plan and should be transparent to the research community.

- Researcher compensation should be linked to successful participation in achieving agreed upon research goals, defined in collaboration with faculty.

5. It is necessary and important to take a collective, institutionwide interest in the time-honored values of the university vis-à-vis learning, investigation, and social responsibility.

- Issues that the study committee have found of increasing concern are (1) excessive and unnecessary faculty secrecy regarding their own research results; (2) individual and institutional conflicts of commitment and interest and; (3) the education of young scientists and conflicts of interest for mentors concerning the value of low-wage, highly productive laboratory assistance provided by their students. None of these issues has an easy answer, but all need ongoing, thoughtful attention by the entire research community at each institution.

6. Necessary capital investments in information systems must be planned for and made in the near term in order to move toward an electronic grant application system capable of incorporating the myriad compliance and accountability steps required by public and private funders and capable of interfacing with an equally modern financial information system.

- This reconfiguring of the electronic infrastructure may be more difficult in the older, larger, more established, and already more fragmented research organizations, but it is an important step in maximizing the delicate balance between functions that must be carried out centrally and decentralized operational capability, responsibility, and accountability.

Patient Care Services: Observations

1. Restructuring the clinical enterprise may alter the distribution of power between the chief executive officer of the academic health center and the president of the parent university.

- When the CEO of the academic health center assumes or is delegated a significant management role in an entity formed through merger or joint operating agreement, that CEO's political leverage, both formal and informal, may be increased relative to that of the president. Conversely, when the clinical enterprise is separated or distanced in a manner that reduces the span of control or budgetary authority of the

CEO of the academic health center, that role may be seen as less powerful in terms of influence within the university. In addition, there is potential for conflict between the CEO of the academic health center and the university president with regard to their respective roles in the governance of a merged entity. In many instances, the university president is on the clinical system board, eclipsing the usual role for a traditional vice president for health affairs.

2. *Urgency to "complete the deal" and work out details later is common and often driven by market forces. A realistic, thorough appraisal of potential consequences before an agreement is signed promotes commitment within the academic health center and creates the possibility to minimize adverse effects. This appraisal process can occur concurrent with due diligence.*

- Restructuring to form joint ventures in clinical services between hospital/health system and the faculty group practice can break down barriers and increase the focus on value (the balance between quality and cost).

3. *It is too early to measure the success of any recent restructuring of the clinical enterprise in academic health centers. At present, most academic health centers are surviving and many are competing very well. Despite this early competitive success, ratcheting down continues. The Balanced Budget Act of 1997, for example, threatens to eliminate for many teaching institutions any prospect for a positive bottom line.*

- Some immediate financial savings can be gained from restructuring the clinical enterprise, but an improved competitive position depends on a number of factors, including careful use of resources, monitoring utilization, appropriate service line consolidation, effective case management, sustained attention to customer satisfaction, and flexibility to meet changing requirements of large managed care payers.
- The impact on educational programs must be monitored over time and can be dramatically affected by service line consolidation, degree of integration of community practice physicians, and amount of weight given to education in determining priorities and practices for the clinical enterprise. The pull of money will need to be countered by

other incentives that promote sustained commitment to the education mission. Similarly, the continued development of research, especially clinical research, will require more than dollars. The willingness of the governance and management of the clinical enterprise to maintain a milieu that fosters clinical research is essential.

4. The tension between university teaching hospitals and their parent universities is altered but not eliminated when the clinical enterprise is separated. University-wide purchasing, contracting, and personnel policies are increasingly a poor fit for academic health centers, which must live in the competitive clinical environment. Separation of the clinical enterprise has an immediate economic impact that benefits the clinical enterprise but may cause tension with the parent university if hospital subsidy of university support systems existed and is suddenly withdrawn.

- For competition in health care delivery, the governance structure must permit optimal functioning of patient care operations, including administrative support. The growing business emphasis on boundary management conflicts with the tight control in many universities.

- Access to capital to purchase sophisticated information systems, to modernize aging facilities, and/or to develop primary care networks is an important requirement for maintaining a competitive position. Distance from the university may improve the academic health center's ability to acquire capital but may adversely affect the university's financial position.

- Conversion of a public academic health center or university hospital to a public corporation may provide direct access to the legislature, a benefit for the academic health center and a source of potential conflict with the parent university.

- The economics of support services and the financial relationship between the academic health center and its parent university change as a result of the shift in operating scale created by the separation. The loss of hospital/health system subsidy of support services may create significant tension within the academic health center or between the academic health center and university.

- With any merger (asset or virtual) some immediate economies of scale can be achieved through consolidation of administrative support services. Centralization is not always the best option as local conditions may override the efficiencies of centralization.

- Organization change is not accomplished simply by an act of merger. Therefore, a well-defined postmerger process should be put in place.

- The transfer of former academic health center employees to new clinical enterprises creates a need for the parent university to support bridging mechanisms in benefits and other human resource programs.

- Unless there is a clear understanding by all parties of the impact of separation of the clinical enterprise on the institution's bonding capacity and fund-raising activities, these issues can generate significant tension within the academic health center and/or between the academic health center and the parent university.

- Care must be taken to protect against the potential loss of the transparent collaboration with parent university/academic health center faculty, the easy use of research facilities, and other university/academic health center resources.

5. *Too little attention is being paid to the complex issues of "organizational culture" in efforts to restructure the clinical enterprise. The task of culture building is enormous and requires a long period of planned intervention and realignment of reward systems.*

- There is extensive evidence from the literature that mergers in health care and other industries rise or fall on the basis of culture. In recounting their own lessons learned, those who report about institutional mergers commonly say they wish they had paid more attention to culture early in the process.

- The cultures of organizations may have common elements but always have points of significant difference. Cultural assessment should be part of due diligence in any actual or virtual merger or any sale.

- Careful analysis of strategic educational needs and clinical business needs and the degree of congruence or conflict between the two is essential in the evaluation of the cultural "fit" between the academic health center and its potential partners.

- Even in the best of circumstances, it takes a long time for people to move from allegiance to a single institution to a system focus. To promote system allegiance, powers should be distributed among the central organization and the individual entities. Each entity and each entity CEO should have systemwide responsibilities.

- Most centers have included only the physicians in their clinical strategic planning, effectively widening the gap separating the health professions from each other and damaging the team-building gestalt.

6. Separation of the clinical enterprise has significant impact on governance. The new governance structure is pulled in the direction of the clinical business and away from the academic missions.

- New governance structures for the clinical enterprise are pulled toward clinical delivery because of the financial magnitude of that enterprise, often without appropriate attention by the governing board to issues affecting education and research. Some lay governance group that could bridge the interface between academic and clinical delivery domains would be useful to support the academic missions.

- For significant and arduous change to occur, the academic health center, university, and trustee leadership must be fully supportive of the plan and the operating leadership. Governance, planning, and capital formation must be completely aligned.

- The CEO of an academic health center who is also in a leadership position of an integrated delivery system is in a fiduciary position for two organizations whose goals and values may be contradictory. Thus is created the potential for awkward situations, misunderstanding, and conflict of interest. Leaders must balance these tensions against the need to integrate across mission areas.

Patient Care Services: Conclusions and Recommendations

1. There is no single best strategy for restructuring the clinical enterprises of academic health centers. Each institution's strategy must be linked to the specific context of the academic health center and the unique demands and opportunities in its environment. Local factors, including institutional resources, competi-

tive environment, political climate, relationship with the practitioner communi-
ty, ownership, governance support, and readiness for change are critical
considerations.

- Successful restructuring requires a partnership between faculty and administration, with deep attention to the present and future quality of student learning, care of patients, and climate for discovery.

- Clinical partnerships and mergers are facilitated when there is a common perception of complementary markets and strengths, and a shared recognition of mutual need and opportunity for benefit through a closer relationship. Mistrust runs deep between academic health centers and community hospitals/health systems. Successful partnerships require a demonstration of commitment to shared goals from both parties.

- A joining of equals is preferable to an apparent takeover by one party. A merger structure with equal voice in governance and equal share in the bottom line for all major parties promotes a sense of willing partners and reduces disputes.

- Changes in leadership create opportunities for new relationships. Several mergers were consummated between previously unwilling partners when one CEO position was vacated. Such opportunities are often more about power than personalities.

- Mergers can be accomplished in the absence of a crisis or sense of urgency, but it requires intense and persistent work to develop and maintain clarity of vision and goals.

- Critical provisions, such as support for the academic missions, dispute mechanisms, buy-back options, and exit conditions, should be covered in the initial formal agreement. The merger guide developed by the University HealthSystem Consortium is a useful outline of critical elements that should be considered.

- The best leverage for negotiating financial support from a clinical partner for the academic missions is before the deal is signed. Educational costs are not well understood, making it difficult to develop a stand-alone rationale for continued support. Analyzing the flow of funds within the academic health center can enhance the academic health center's bargaining position.

- The clearer and more realistic the academic health center is on what it can deliver in a partnership or merger, the stronger the negotiating position. The academic health center's negotiating power in new academic and clinical environments may be enhanced by a better organization of institutional medicine, such as contracts with state agencies for outsourced services that the academic health center may be uniquely positioned to deliver.

2. Attention must be given to some strong structural balance that ensures appropriate attention to education and research and thereby counter any tendency of the new clinical entity to migrate away from the academic missions.

- The academic health center cannot expect its CEO to single-handedly carry its agenda in dealings with an integrated delivery system, regardless of the leverage an academic health center might have. This emerging executive responsibility requires support from university administration, department chairs, and faculty; a core group must have received preparation in skills of advanced executive leadership (finance and high-level negotiation).

- Physicians and other health professionals must be actively involved in every level of governance and management of the clinical enterprise to garner their support. Physicians must be willing to develop the necessary skills and assume appropriate accountability. Although nursing schools have paid much attention to the development of administrative skills among their faculty, as yet, there seems to be only a small pool of faculty physicians prepared for significant roles in system governance or management.

3. The reality of the market requires academic health centers to compete on price in order to sustain a patient base adequate to the needs of the academic program. Unless academic health centers apply sound business principles to the structure and management of clinical services, they are unlikely to be successful competitors in health care delivery.

- Faculty practice groups are migrating from federations of distinct department or division-based plans to unified plans with centralized governance and financial management. Progress is slow in migration to a true seamless group practice that is oriented to the success of the entire institution.

- To ensure viability of the academic health center, the clinical enterprise must be consolidated as a single entity, managed according to sound business principles, and focused on the strategic priorities of the entire academic health center. Continued fragmentation of effort along departmental lines is contrary to financial and program success of the whole.

- The CEO of the academic health center must have, either directly or indirectly, the ability to focus the entire clinical enterprise on strategic priorities of the institution, the authority to commit resources and people, and the capacity to deliver on commitments.

- The ability to contract as an institution with state agencies, corporations, or foreign entities for services strengthens the competitive position of the academic health center.

- Long-term linkage of the clinical enterprise to the academic missions cannot be left to chance or good will. It must be ensured, either through ownership by the academic health center or contractual agreement with a non-owned or mutually owned health system.

4. *Institutions may underestimate the leverage clinical research can provide in crafting a clinical partnership, particularly if the academic health center's focus is on basic science research.*

- The value of clinical research as a means to maintain competitive advantage is sound justification for investment of health system funds in research and may also be a mechanism for bringing faculty and community physicians together in a joint effort.

- Although price currently drives the system, academic health centers should attempt to lead in quality measurements innovation and clinical evaluation.

5. *The metrics for managing the interface between academics and the service system are deficient and must be improved. The clients or the people to be served are the individual patients and the relevant population. Patient outcomes and health status markers for the whole population, including proper surrogate measures for desirable results of care, are at the core of a proper evaluation system.*

EPILOGUE

1. The relationship between the academic health center and its community—city, state, or region—is a critical leverage point as the academic health center undergoes transformational change. Perceptions of how well the academic health center meets important health needs of the local community can facilitate or sidetrack efforts by the academic health center to create partnerships, increase cost effectiveness, reshape the workforce, introduce new products, or modify the class sizes or composition of health professions schools.

- Perceptions of how well an academic health center serves critical health needs of the local community have greater political impact as resources are constrained. More academic health centers are developing or extending relationships with their community, both out of a sense of mission and to cultivate public support.

- With increasing penetration of managed care plans and other cost containment strategies, academic health centers and other local health care providers have a common interest in keeping the local population healthy. Ideally, this should be a common effort in order to provide a comprehensive and nonduplicative health promotion strategy for the community.

- With the shift of health care practice to ambulatory settings, academic health centers are increasingly reliant on affiliations and other relationships with a broad array of community providers, both institutional and individual.

- The local community can be an important market for introduction of new educational products or clinical services. In addition, a number of academic health center business services could be expanded to local customers to enhance revenue.

- Almost half of member institutions of the Association of Academic Health Centers (AHC) have established a health policy and/or health services research center. The committee recommends that more institutions follow suit because such centers can help stimulate public discussion on the increasing number of societal and policy conundrums we shall need to confront.

2. *Education of the public is an increasingly important role for academic health centers.* As we strive to make health care more patient-centered, patients have a critical need for information about health, illness, and treatment options in order to participate meaningfully in their care. As part of their community service mission, academic health centers should be providing access to the very best such information available.

3. *Schools and programs in public health and departments of community and family medicine, epidemiology, community and public health nursing, and dentistry are increasingly important assets for academic health centers in their community relationships and activities.* Expertise in these areas should be appropriately harnessed to serve community health needs, track population measures of health status, and develop health promotion and disease prevention programs in conjunction with community and public health agencies.

4. *Public support for research is challenged both in terms of level of support and disease-specific direction of funds.* It is in the academic health center's interest to promote greater public understanding of the benefits that accrue to society from basic and clinical research in order to facilitate a consistent level of public funding. Outreach education efforts, "mini-medical school" programs for the public, presentations to civic groups, and relationships with K–12 school systems can foster a public understanding of science.

5. *A recent AHC member survey shows that more than half have significant international activities, demonstrating that the community is now in fact global in dimension, even as it remains local and regional in its most intense focus.*

6. *The committee noted that the recent changes in direction of the health care system of the U.S. Department of Veterans Affairs (VA) and its associated multiprofessional clinical education programs should make the VA an even more important partner for its associated academic health centers.* Moreover, in an era of cost constraint that will probably continue to encroach on resources for the academic missions, affiliations between the VA and health professions schools provide new and expanded opportunities for innovative health professions curriculum development and patient-focused research.

7. *To ensure that the community is well served by the academic health center as*

a whole, it is recommended that there be a central academic health center office that keeps track of and coordinates, if it does not manage, institutional programs in the community. To address the international community, most academic health centers may opt to create a separate central venue.

In summary, the scientific opportunities for academic health centers have never been greater, but the financial stringencies have never been more threatening. For these institutions to successfully bring education, research, and patient care together in new configurations that capitalize on today's revolution in science, serve the community, and remain true to their core university values will require strong and visionary leadership, well-informed and flexible governance, and an educated and committed public. In the long run, the success of any particular adaptation will depend on each individual academic health center's anatomy, physiology, culture, and local environment.

CHAPTER 1

MINDING THE
TRIPARTITE MISSION

Elaine R. Rubin, PhD

O VER THE PAST FEW YEARS, ACADEMIC HEALTH centers have been employing a number of strategies to respond to current market forces and enhance their competitiveness in the clinical service arena. The focus of most of the discussion has been on establishing mechanisms to reduce costs and increase productivity and efficiency in hospital and other patient-care clinical services; the measures have included downsizing staff, consolidating clinical services, and modifying decision-making processes structures.

Less attention, however, has been devoted to the many other activities already underway to reshape the academic responsibilities—that is, the education and research missions—of the academic health centers. Indeed, many leaders of academic health centers have been voicing concerns for some time about a range of organizational, governance, and management issues prompted by the new environment that have broad implications not only for health care but also for the higher education community.

The Association of Academic Health Centers (AHC) recognizes that such concerns suggest that academic health centers, like similar institutions with changing societal roles that go beyond economic goals, may be showing the symptoms of age. In light of such concerns, both the public ideals and demands that created and sustained the institutions require reexamination.

Dr. Rubin is the assistant vice president for program of the Association of Academic Health Centers.

Over the past two years, therefore, the AHC has published several reports in the form of case studies on the response of various centers to the new health care environment. Based on presentations by members at various AHC meetings and symposia, these case studies are here gathered together for the first time in a single publication (appendix A). These firsthand accounts of change underway within a number of AHC member institutions are not intended to be detailed, analytical institutional reviews. But as individual snapshots of change taking place at some academic health centers, they highlight some distinguishing variables and particular aspects of change at these institutions, including the institutional environment and the strategic planning, recent restructuring, change processes, innovative programs, new partnerships, and leadership interventions occurring in different locales.

Thus, in an area where little literature is available and anecdotal evidence is abundant, the case studies help to fill a void by providing concrete information on some of the key issues confronting academic health centers today.

OVERVIEW

Taken together, the case studies reveal a situation at odds with the stereotypical view of institutions out of touch with rapidly evolving environments. Instead, the cases reveal institutions that are major forces in local or regional economies and that are taking proactive measures to respond to change. The modifications that have taken place at these institutions appear, in turn, to have created and encouraged an atmosphere conducive to reassessment of the nature and relevance of the academic health center, its missions, and its functions.

In general, and as in most of the literature, clinical issues and financial concerns tend to dominate the discussions in the case studies because, for the most part, these issues have been and continue to be the major catalysts of institutional change. However, the interconnection of the service mission with the education and research missions is revealed in the other themes that emerge from the papers, including reappraisal of the academic mission, reexaminination of cultures and values when institutions reshape the functions, transformation in organization and governance, and evolution in the nature of leadership.

The future, of course, depends a great deal on how institutions respond to changing economics. For example, the loss of the ability to support education and research through funds that flowed from the clinical enterprise is a fundamental issue that institutions are now addressing. But academic health center leaders are recognizing that they must look beyond economics and the health care environment to consider and confront higher education where societal expectations and demands for accountability are mounting. These papers raise awareness about how dependent and interrelated these two worlds are.

Although all the cases do not explicitly address academic issues, concern for the viability of the education and research missions lies at the heart of much of the discussions of the situation in which the clinical enterprise finds itself. The Creighton University study, for example, examines the difficulties the university encountered in attempting to preserve its education mission after the sale of St. Joseph Hospital, its major teaching affiliate. Studies from the Cornell University Medical College and the University of Texas Southwestern Medical Center at Dallas focus on the challenge of sustaining a research enterprise as well as the strategies and innovative approaches being taken to underwrite research activities. And the study of the merger of the Pennsylvania State University and the Geisinger Health System describes Penn State's strategy to seek a partnership that would preserve and enhance its educational and research missions. The merged health care system that was developed recognized the importance of these missions through the creation and maintenance of an academic support formula that would provide funds to the Pennsylvania State University College of Medicine.

Such cases pay particular attention to the research enterprise, which is in a critical stage of transition within academic health centers. Clinical research is particularly vulnerable as academic health centers are constrained by the loss of patient care revenues from Medicare, Medicaid, and the private market. The financial challenges facing the academic health centers, which have led the way in nurturing and supporting biomedical research since the end of World War II, now have less capacity to put together the patchwork of institutional funds, revenues from patient care, and grants from public and private sources that traditionally supported research. Research funding, in and of itself, is usually not sufficient to cover total research costs. Indirect costs, faculty recruitment costs, training costs, and costs incurred to meet federal and state compliance standards are not always fully reimbursed but nevertheless must be factored into maintaining the enterprise.

An increased focus on strategic planning that includes organizational design, revenue distribution, networking, and development strategies is a theme that runs throughout the studies that follow. Strategic planning receives attention in the University of Illinois at Chicago case, which examines the key factors that have shaped a public university's perceptions about the academic health center and the management and organization of the institution in recent years.

The study of Rush-Presbyterian-St. Luke's Medical Center recounts a strategic planning initiative dating back to 1984 that sought to develop options for one of the earliest vertically integrated health systems. This study illustrates the creative visions and philosophies that helped build the institutions, as well as the unique corporate and governance structures that evolved. In central Pennsylvania, leaders of Penn State's College of Medicine noted the rapid growth of market-driven health care reform in the early 1990s and foresaw that the institutional missions could be threatened by remaining isolated in the market. Therefore, they began a purposeful quest to join with an institution of similar history, culture, and mission. The Penn State Geisinger Health System resulted from the work of leaders and others throughout both organizations who were able to look beyond the status quo to transform institutions for the future. The outcomes of institutional strategic planning, including the creation of centers of excellence, point to a highly individualized approach to change that is a central and recurrent theme of these and other studies of academic health centers nationwide.

The study from the Medical College of Wisconsin outlines a strategic plan that includes efforts to increase primary care capacity, reduce costs, and develop advanced information systems in a highly competitive market environment. The case of Wake Forest University School of Medicine (formerly Wake Forest/ Bowman Gray School of Medicine) emphasizes information technology and describes its critical function within the institution's strategic plan.

The evolution in the organization and governance of institutions and the search for autonomy, particularly in public institutions, is detailed in the case from Oregon Health Sciences University (OHSU). The Tulane University case examines the economic environment and the decisions that led to the sale of the Tulane University Hospital to Columbia/HCA, an investor-owned corporation. Detail on the governance of the new company that formed as a result of the sale is provided, along with discussion of the implications for education and research. In its efforts to preserve the academic mission, Wake Forest University School of

Medicine selected a dual strategy of change targeted at both internal and external organizational structures. The case study outlines the strategy and provides a detailed look at some of the outcomes in an institution with a centralized governance and organizational structures and a unique historical relationship with its primary affiliated teaching hospital and the practicing physicians in the community.

Finally, the case from the Western University of Health Sciences describes new educational strategies, structures, and programs that evolved in the period when the institution was transformed from the College of Osteopathic Medicine of the Pacific to the Western University of Health Sciences.

CASE STUDY HIGHLIGHTS

Numerous lessons can be extrapolated from the case studies. Many echo findings from studies of academic health centers by other major organizations and consulting firms. But the lessons bear repeating because they remain critical variables to understanding and managing change and reconfiguration for the future. Perhaps the most important lesson that emerges is that cookie-cutter solutions cannot be applied to academic health centers. Each institution remains a unique product of its history, culture, and environment. Some case study highlights follow.

The Changing Nature of Leadership

The roles, responsibilities, and relationships of academic health center and university leaders have long been viewed as significant aspects of the organization and governance of academic health centers. Strong, effective leadership appears as a given in describing what makes organizations function well and successfully. Of late, much has been written about what characteristics distinguish a leader, the nature of leadership, and the evolution in the types and character of organizational leaders. Many theories and studies of organizations and change have also focused on the leader's ability to generate and implement change and take an active role in the creation of organizational culture. The visions of leaders, their rhetoric, and their ability to communicate with others can be major factors in determining institutional success or failure. Such theories are quite relevant for academic health centers confronting or undergoing change. As some of the studies suggest, new and different management skills are required to lead academic health centers. Leaders are also balancing priorities, exercising authority, and using communication skills and technologies in new and different ways.

Creating Environments for Change

- The most important characteristic of a good leader is the ability to create readiness for change and an understanding of the change processes.

All the case studies point to leadership as the critical variable in managing change. The case study of Wake Forest University School of Medicine, for example, illustrates how important it is for a leader not only to articulate a vision for the institution but also to understand the academic and institutional cultures. "Change does not occur without acceptance by the people who are doing the work," says Richard Janeway, MD, the then executive vice president for health affairs at Wake Forest University and chief executive officer of the Bowman Gray School of Medicine. Notes Janeway, "The 'suits' cannot force change."

Keeping Constituencies Informed

- Leaders must place a premium on communication to keep faculty, staff, and students informed, particularly where new and complex arrangements, affiliations, or mergers are being negotiated or before all aspects of an arrangement are made public.
- The centralization of decision-making power has intensified the need to communicate; at the same time, it has created a major problem about defining the message, that is, how and what to communicate with administrators and faculty, many of whom may now have diminished powers in the organization.
- Involvement of governing boards and faculty on strategic issues related to operations, health professions, research, health care delivery, and the faculty practice plan is a key to ensuring buy-in to planned changes.

The case studies view communication as critical in times of organizational change. The Tulane and Creighton studies are most significant in this regard, given their merger with large for-profit enterprises with cultures that in many ways were perceived as diametrically opposed to the academic and nonprofit worlds.

They point out the need for keeping faculty, staff, and community leaders informed when major mergers, sales of facilities, or corporate restructuring are under consideration. In analyzing the Penn State Geisinger Health System merger, Dr. C. McCollister Evarts made note that throughout months of confidential planning and negotiations, the leadership of both organizations participated fully in the process.

Extending Development Efforts

- Institutional leaders are placing increased emphasis on development efforts.
- Philanthropic support, particularly major gifts from private donors, is being used by some institutions as a major strategy for generating research support.

The experience of the University of Texas Southwestern Medical Center at Dallas highlights the changing environment for development, with the university shifting some of its efforts from the grateful patient as donor to local foundations, businesses, and individuals whose primary motives for giving are general altruism, the desire to conquer disease, and civic pride. The university has also capitalized on its image as the only "world class" medical institution in Dallas. The one-person development office in 1985 has grown into a twelve-person office with a budget of $600,000. Total philanthropic support was $49.2 million in 1995, with more than $30 million coming from the community.

Increased reliance on philanthropy to support research will require that institutions identify new sources of funds to cover indirect costs that are not covered by private gifts. The University of Texas Southwestern Medical Center at Dallas case provides valuable information about development strategies and activities.

Enabling Quick Response

- Institutional leaders must have authority.

Several of the studies, including those from the Rush-Presbyterian-St. Luke's Medical Center and the Medical College of Wisconsin, point out the importance of having leaders with decision-making authority and structures that permit rapid decision-making. Some institutions are also centralizing decision-making processes related to the allocation of resources for facilities and programs, which often includes designating one executive with powers to control all investment dollars.

At the University of Illinois at Chicago (UIC), the vice chancellor for health services controls such investment dollars (other than the dean's tax) for the clinical enterprise. Faculty recruitment or development of new facilities and programs (which are aligned with strategic development goals) cannot go forward without the vice chancellor's approval.

Centralization of Decision-making

- Centralized governance and management structures can permit rapid decision-making in today's health care market.
- The governance structure must permit optimal functioning of service operations.
- Strategic planning as well as urgent planning is needed to permit rapid decision-making.
- Drawing clinical leadership into governance and management can be a major factor in breaking down barriers between administrative and clinical structures.

Academic health centers are increasingly streamlining or centralizing decision-making mechanisms and processes in order to respond rapidly to market conditions. Some are doing both.

The Wake Forest University School of Medicine and the UIC studies highlight the university's centralized governance structure and how centralized governance provides flexibility in medical school decisionmaking.

The Rush-Presbyterian-St. Luke's Medical Center case describes highly centralized and controlled governance and management structures that oversee operations of very complex organizations and corporate activities.

The University of Illinois at Chicago case points to the restructuring of its clinics as joint ventures between the hospital and medical service plans as one way to break down barriers between hospital administration and clinician structures.

Access to Capital

- For all academic health centers, whether public or private, access to capital is critical to modernize aging facilities and equipment and to develop a health system or network.

Public academic health centers are often hampered by state contracting, purchasing, and personnel rules, which do not permit the institutions to make a timely response to a rapidly changing health care environment. Some institutions are seeking freedom from cumbersome state governance structures so that their primary teaching-hospital function can function more effectively and efficiently and to have easier access to capital.

The OHSU experience shows that the conversion of a public academic health center from a state agency to a public corporation resulted in a streamlined, centralized decision-making structure with governance of the institution by a single, independent board. Conversion enhanced the ability of the institution to compete in the clinical service arena and also increased access to the state legislature by permitting the institution to provide direct testimony on appropriations and other issues.

Like many universities, OHSU was also seeking easier access to capital to modernize its plant and equipment. Access to the bond markets was dependent on the state, with the university usually part of a larger state bond package that pitted its needs against those of other unrelated state functions. A growing $120+ million deferred maintenance problem was one catalyst for becoming a public corporation.

Governance

- Strong local governance can be an issue in a merger of an academic health center teaching hospital with a large health system, particularly a for-profit system.

Strong local governance of St. Joseph Hospital, Creighton University's teaching hospital, was an important part of Creighton's negotiating stance when the hospital was acquired by American Medical International (AMI), an investor-owned, for-profit company. Local governance became an issue of conflict when AMI changed ownership and was one reason Creighton explored its buyback option. Creighton officials particularly noted the importance of strong local governance in academic health center-corporate relations. The community, they point out in their case study, not only must support and defend the academic health center tripartite mission but also must help to ensure that the hospital, in particular, operates to meet local needs.

In the Penn State Geisinger Health System merger, two nonprofit enterprises with similar histories and cultures created a single governance structure. The appointment of an executive leadership team, as well as appointments of leaders of the health system, clinical divisions, and the corporate office were considered among the postmerger accomplishments.

Culture

- Cultural factors within and among organizations often become paramount in designing and implementing organizational change. Within academic health centers, the ascendance of the entrepreneurial outlook has created tensions and conflict within the academic world. Cultural differences also emerge in relationships between academic health centers and other not-for-profit organizations.
- The cultural problems of mergers are great unless institutions with similar missions share common values.
- Faculty morale can pose difficulty in times of mergers, sales, or other changes in ownership or governance of the clinical enterprise.
- Clinical faculty between the ages of 40 and 55 may generate the most anger against change within a system because the anticipated promises of rewards from the system have not been realized.

The Tulane and Creighton cases emphasize the critical nature of the cultural match in mergers of academic health centers with for-profit health care enterprises. The Cornell University Medical College case study highlights institutional and faculty culture vis-à-vis organizational changes that are unrelated to sales or mergers. The Cornell study notes the critical significance of faculty attitudes when considering changes in the structure of the practice plan. The Penn State Geisinger Health System highlights the cultural similarities of the two organizations but nevertheless points out that long-term success will depend on the ability to recognize existing cultures while still creating and layering a new organizational culture over them.

Education and Research

- In any merger, the educational and research requirements for the academic health center must be agreed upon early in the negotiation process. The obligations related to support for graduate medical education must be clearly defined.
- Promoting and sustaining the academic health center mission in dealings with health systems of which the academic health center is a part can require tremendous time and effort in light of the frequent changes in management that often occur in corporate structures.
- Academic health centers are increasingly seeking to align the institution's clinical and academic networks.
- The size and costs of educational programs are key items on the academic health center agenda for the future.
- The expansion and use of information systems will be essential to success.

The Tulane, Creighton, and Penn State cases provide the greatest detail on merger issues. The University of Illinois at Chicago case describes the institution's efforts to achieve its goal of focusing its academic resources on a limited number of partners and exploiting these academic relationships in clinical business relationships. The UIC and Cornell studies raise the complex issue of determining the costs of health professions education.

Technology Transfer

- Academic health centers are seeking to maximize money earned through technology transfer agreements and royalties.

The case study from the University of Texas Southwestern Medical Center at Dallas highlights both the problems and the potential of technology transfer activities. Although many institutions have pursued technology transfer quite vigorously, the activities have proved only modestly successful as a way to cross-subsidize research. Significant funds are usually generated by only a few laboratories. The Gatorade experience, where a discovery results in enormous profits being returned to the university, is rare.

Research Space

- There is a clear trend toward centralizing the way research space is allocated within the academic health center.
- There are some indications of a breakdown of the departmental basis for instruction in medical schools; to encourage cross-subsidization of basic sciences, for example, linkages are taking place between the basic sciences and clinical departments.

The Cornell University Medical College case reveals a cross-subsidization of basic sciences occurring through marriages of shared interests rather than fund transfers (e.g., pharmacology and anesthesiology). It is one example of attempts to break down departmental boundaries. In addition, Cornell's neuroscience program, rather than remaining a free-standing program or department, is now embedded in the neurology and psychiatry departments.

Curricular Change

- Periods of organizational transformation can bode well for making fundamental changes in curricula, the physical design of educational facilities, the departmental structure, and faculty roles.

The case study of Western University of Health Sciences reveals that periods of change can provide opportunities to design a new educational environment. In its transition from a college to a university, leaders expanded institutional priorities to include integration of humanism into the campus community, establishment of multidisciplinary health professions programs, and evaluation of societal issues related to health and disease. Innovative learning methods, such as using interactive technologies, were implemented when the university established a new College of Pharmacy. The architectural design of the college optimized structures and configurations that were conducive to collaboration and interaction among students, faculty, and administrators.

Financing Research

- Some academic health centers have lost almost all of their capacity to subsidize research from clinical profits; these institutions assume that the faculty practice plan can no longer serve as a major way to underwrite research activities.

The University of Texas Southwestern Medical Center at Dallas and the Cornell University Medical College studies focus particular attention on this issue. The Texas study notes, for example, that in 1985, sources of seed money to initiate new research programs and to support young investigators came primarily from general and institutional state appropriations (as opposed to funds explicitly appropriated for research).

Centers of Excellence

- Centers of Excellence are a means to raise the research profile of the institution and to realign power and organizational relationships. To some degree, they are also a marketing tool, projecting a cuttinge-edge research image to the public.

The Rush case study points to a strategic plan that designed a number of centers of excellence as a way to demonstrate institutional commitment to research as well as patient care. The centers reflect a multidisciplinary approach to research and patient care.

Researchers

- The profile of investigators being recruited to academic health centers is undergoing major change.

The Cornell University Medical College case is a study of how institutions are reexamining their recruitment profiles and strategies in the biomedical sciences. The profile of investigators who are considered to be good investments for venture capital initiatives has changed, for example. Institutions are now concentrating on recruiting only A+ investigators, thus creating a possibly shrinking job market for graduates in the basic sciences.

Public Commitments

- Academic health centers not only have retained their traditional mission of service to the poor at increasingly great expense but are also renewing or taking on community commitments that include service and education.
- Academic health centers are undertaking initiatives to increase their power and effectiveness in state relations.

- Academic health centers are increasing initiatives to educate state policy-makers about the value of academic medicine.

Many of the case studies note an increase in their legislative involvement at the state level, a situation that may reflect, in part, a shift in powers and authorities from the Federal government to the states in the health care arena.

Academic health centers increasingly perceive a need to educate public policy-makers and other local and institutional decision-makers about health issues. These issues include the impact of competition on academic health centers, the value of academic medicine, the economic impact of individual institutions within a state, and the need to preserve the academic health center education and research mission. Often, academic health centers have taken the lead in forming coalitions to address such concerns. The University of Illinois at Chicago case study calls attention to public policy issues and reveals how the institution's efforts resulted in increased state appropriations.

MODELS FOR THE FUTURE

The studies, intended from the start to showcase positive strategies and actions with potential for replication, do not always highlight the inevitable problems, conflicts, and controversies encountered along the way to success. However, in addressing the academic mission specifically, they raise questions about societal interests and responsibilities as health professions education and research reach beyond the institution to benefit people throughout the world. In this way, the cases can contribute to a better understanding of the ways that academic health centers are seeking to redefine and preserve their special functions, roles, and values in a rapidly changing world.

CHAPTER 2

THE EVOLVING STRUCTURE, ORGANIZATION, AND GOVERNANCE OF ACADEMIC HEALTH CENTERS

Marian Osterweis, PhD

A S PART OF THE ASSOCIATION OF ACADEMIC Health Centers (AHC) study on the response of academic health centers to the rapid and dramatic evolution occurring in both the health care marketplace and the financing of health services, the Study Committee supplemented its case studies and site visits with a mail survey of all 99 of AHC member institutions. Questions focused primarily on changes in overall organization, structure, and governance in the period 1997–1998, particularly as they relate to the mission areas of education, research, and clinical services. Appendix B contains the questionnaire.

The overwhelming impression from the findings, which, in essence, provide a representative sample of the universe of academic health centers, is that many institutions are making profound, creative changes in every aspect of operations so that they can cope with the new health care environment while continuing to serve their communities.

This trend was first noted by the AHC in 1992 and again in 1994 when AHC surveyed its membership on matters relating to the growth of managed care, changing health care delivery systems, the workforce, and academic health center–university relations. Indeed, because a number of key questions have been repeated over the years, the results of the three surveys are beginning to

---

Dr. Osterweis is executive vice president of the Association of Academic Health Centers.

yield a longitudinal view of the adjustments that academic health centers are making in response to growing pressures from many sources. And, as in the past, no single model of an academic health center emerged. Instead, local conditions and historical patterns, coupled with individual leadership strengths and concerns, continue to influence the shape of the institutions.

METHODOLOGY

The questions for the 1997–1998 survey were designed to gather mostly qualitative information in the following six areas.

1. Scope of responsibility and authority of the academic health center leaders.
2. Institutional flexibility, as evidenced by contracting authority, the availability of funds, and mechanisms for raising capital.
3. Governance of the academic health center, its parent university, and one or more health-system components, including changes in the previous year.
4. Funding, organization, sizing, and reward systems for health professions education.
5. Research environment, including recent changes in the organization of the research enterprise and relations with industry.
6. Scope and structure of clinical services and changes in the previous year in the patient care components of academic health centers.

Data were examined in light of four control variables that the Study Committee had a priori reason to believe might influence responses.

1. *Public or private status.* In addition to differences in governance structures and procedures, one would generally expect that private institutions have greater flexibility in all aspects of their operations and are able to make changes more easily than public institutions.
2. *University-based, freestanding, or part of a state system.* The presidents and chancellors of the freestanding academic health centers and many state-system institutions are responsible for the entire campus. They would be expected to have more responsibility and authority and therefore greater ability to control and make changes in all areas than the vice presidents who report to university presidents.

3. *Ownership or nonownership of teaching hospital.* Hospital ownership can create special stresses in today's environment, profoundly affecting the finances of the entire academic health center. Such a situation might be expected to cause changes in institutional behavior in an attempt to ensure continued competitiveness in the clinical maketplace.

4. *Managed-care market stage.* In 1992, the University HealthSystem Consortium (UHC) developed a market classification tool incorporating 16 variables (including HMO penetration, insurance premium levels, and level of prepayment to physicians) to define four stages of market development within a geographical area.*

One would predict profound changes in the academic health centers within a specific geographical region as the area moves from stage I (relatively high reimbursement and traditional fee-for-service mechanisms) to the hypercompetition characterizing stage IV markets, in which a few large, integrated providers compete to provide comprehensive services to defined populations in the region. In other words, the greater the managed-care penetration, the greater the financial and operational pressures on the academic health center. As with hospital ownership, one would anticipate that such pressures would result in more organizational changes in every realm.

RESULTS

The overall response rate was 73 percent (72 out of 99), although, as with most surveys, not every respondent answered every question. Survey respondents mirror key characteristics in the universe of academic health centers and AHC membership in terms of institutional type. As shown in table 1, more than half of the respondents are public institutions; over two-thirds are part of comprehensive universities; and about 20 percent are freestanding health science universities. The majority own their primary teaching hospital.

Unfortunately, UHC has not classified every locale in terms of its managed-care market stage. As a result, data are missing for many of the responding

---

*Robert J. Baker, president and chief executive officer of the University HealthSystem Consortium, discusses four distinct stages of market competition and the evolution of the managed care marketplace in volume 2 of *Mission Management: A New Synthesis.*

Table 1.

KEY CHARACTERISTICS OF ACADEMIC HEALTH CENTERS, 1997–98

Characteristic	Survey Respondents (72)	AHC Membership (99)	Universe (124)
Public institution	43 (60%)	56 (57%)	71 (57%)
Private institution	29 (40%)	43 (43%)	53 (43%)
University-based	50 (69%)	65 (66%)	89 (72%)
Freestanding	14 (19%)	23 (23%)	25 (20%)
Part of state system*	8 (11%)	11 (11%)	10 (8%)
Owns hospital	40 (56%)	56 (57%)	NA
Doesn't own hospital	32 (44%)	47 (44%)	NA

* The Association of Academic Health Centers defines a "state system" as a public university system that has an established state office with an executive head of health affairs (currently, California, New York, Texas).

institutions and the broader universe of academic health centers. In addition, where an academic health center has clinical operations in a number of locales (some fairly distant and in different market stages), the center as a whole could not be fairly characterized.

The findings do show, however, that among respondents, 8 institutions (11%) were in stage I; 15 (21%) were in stage II; 23 (32%) were in stage III; 8 (11%) were in stage IV; and 18 (25%) could not be classified.

Institutional leadership. Table 2 shows the titles of the heads of AHC's member institutions. These titles mirror the universe of academic health centers. Almost 40 percent are presidents or chancellors of health sciences campuses, which may be freestanding universities or part of a state university system; another 40 percent are vice presidents or vice chancellors for health affairs, often with another academic title or a title that reflects their role in the health system. Of the remaining 20 percent, most are deans of medicine, usually with another academic title as well. It is interesting to note that some heads of academic health centers who are now also heads of health systems or clinical networks have true corporate chief executive titles. In general, there appears to be a trend toward more multiple titles, including both academic and health system ones.

Table 2.
TITLES OF ACADEMIC HEALTH CENTER LEADERS

Title	Number
President or chancellor	35
President and dean of medicine	3
Subtotal	*38*
Vice president, vice chancellor, or Executive vice president/vice chancellor for health affairs	16
VP and CEO or other title in health system	5
VP or CEO of health system and dean of medicine	2
VP and dean of medicine	13
VP and other	6
Subtotal	*42*
Dean of medicine	3
Dean and other title (not VP), e.g., provost for medical affairs	7
Dean and CEO of health system	2
Subtotal	*12*
CEO of health system only	3
Subtotal	*3*
Other	4
Total	*99*

The heads of academic health centers, regardless of title, have powerful jobs and, according to the most recent survey, there is some evidence that their scope of authority and responsibility has expanded in recent years. For example:

- The vast majority of academic health center heads have direct-line authority over most of the deans of the health professions schools on their campuses (table 3). Those in academic health centers and universities that own their hospital may also have authority over the administrator of the hospital. Since 1992, the percentage with direct authority over the hospital and the schools of nursing, pharmacy, public health, and graduate studies has grown somewhat.
- The great majority of academic health center leaders have direct-line authority for the major institutional support offices, including the key

Table 3.
**PERCENTAGE OF ACADEMIC HEALTH CENTER LEADERS
WITH DIRECT-LINE AUTHORITY OVER VARIOUS DEANS AND DIRECTORS**

School or Component	Percentage	Ratio*
School of allied health	85	33/39
School of dentistry	76	26/34
School of medicine+	95	57/60
School of nursing	86	42/49
School of pharmacy	96	25/26
School of public health	95	20/21
Graduate studies	100	35/35
Hospital	73	30/41

* Number of academic health center leaders with direct authority for a particular school or component, divided by the number of institutions with such a school or component.

+ Non-dean respondents.

offices of development and fund-raising (74%), finance (86%), government relations (71%), human resources (63%), marketing (77%), planning (81%), and public relations (84%). These numbers are up somewhat since 1992.

- Heads of academic health centers who are presidents, chancellors, or vice presidents and the equivalent, are more likely than deans of medicine (with or without another title) to have control over key offices. Not surprisingly, among the 50 university-based respondents, some support positions are shared with the parent university. The offices of directors of development, government relations, human resources, and public relations are most likely to be shared with the parent university (31%, 28%, and 22%, respectively). On the other hand, it is noteworthy that among the university-based respondents, only 4 percent share all the major positions with the university and 22 percent share none.

- Almost all (93%) of the academic health center leaders report that they have access to flexible funds that allow them to initiate new programs and stimulate change in their institution.

- Heads of private institutions, freestanding institutions, and institutions owning their own hospitals report having more flexible funds than their counterparts in other institutions.

- The vast majority of leaders (97%) report having power of the budget, and 72 percent report being able to shift funds from one health professions school to another, up from 59 percent in 1992.
- Among the heads of the freestanding academic health centers, 90 percent are able to shift funds among schools, as compared with only 67 percent in university-based academic health centers.
- Not only do the heads of the academic health centers sit on most major boards of the center, the owned and affiliated clinical entities, and many of the university governing bodies, but they also chair and appoint members to many institutional governing bodies as well. In this way, they at least participate in, and often control, the composition of the governance structures. Even in institutions that have separated their clinical enterprises from the university, the heads of the academic health centers continue to participate in the governance of those entities, thus maintaining formal influence over the clinical operations that continue to be needed for teaching and research.

Institutional flexibility. Single-signature contracting and improved ability to form capital have made many academic health centers more nimble in recent years, and hence better able to compete in the clinical marketplace.

- More than half of the respondents (58) report that the academic health center has single-signature contracting capability; those who own their hospital and are in more advanced market stages are somewhat more likely to have it. Not surprisingly, institutions that are part of a state system are less likely than either university-based or freestanding institutions to have single-signature contracting authority (38% compared with 62% and 60%, respectively).
- The primary mechanisms for capital formation are bonds (66%), gifts (66%), and loans (41%). Gifts and loans are more common among private than public institutions (90% and 69% compared with 50% and 22%). State appropriations are more common among public institutions than private ones (34% vs. 10%). Clinical revenues are mentioned by only 14 percent of the respondents as a way to raise

money, and they are more likely to be mentioned by those who do not own their own hospital rather than by those who do (22% compared with 7%). Asset appreciation and income from investments were mentioned by 23 percent of the respondents.

- Overall, 35 percent of the respondents report that their ability to form capital had changed in the previous two years. Within this group, the majority (64%) say this ability has improved. Those who own their own hospital and are in more advanced market stages are more likely than others to report positive changes in capital formation. Most (80%) report that their institutions are allowed to acquire debt. Those who own a hospital are more likely to be able to acquire debt than those who do not own a hospital (89% compared with 69%).

- It came as somewhat a surprise to the study team to discover that half the respondents report they have adequate capital to meet their education, research, and clinical service goals. Respondents from private institutions (55%), freestanding academic health centers (86%), and institutions that do not own a hospital (56%) were more likely than their counterparts in other institutions to say they had adequate capital.

- Asked about contracts with their parent university or university systems for such services as security and maintenance, the vast majority (81%) report that no changes occurred in the previous year.

Governance. Several significant conclusions can be drawn from the series of questions regarding governance. First, academic health center governance is highly variable. Second, especially among public institutions, governance is not controlled by the academic health center or its parent university (if there is one). Third, governance structures of the academic health centers and their clinical services are changing. More specifically:

- Academic health center governing bodies are most often appointed (79%), especially among public institutions (90%) where the governor is the primary person to make the appointments. Elected and self-perpetuating boards are more common in private institutions than in public ones (38% and 41% compared with 15% and 2%, respectively). Seventeen percent of institutions use multiple methods to make appointments to the board.

- Only 19 (26%) of the respondents report that the academic health center has its own governing board, and 50 (68%) report that the center is governed by a university or university-system board. One-third of the latter group said that a subset of the board has true governing authority over the center.

- About half the respondents have a separate health-system or clinical network governing board. Private, university-based institutions that own their own hospitals are more likely than others to have health-system boards.

- Overall, 44 percent report having a visiting committee of external advisors.

- Changes in the governance structures of academic health centers in the previous year are reported by 29 percent of the respondents, and 44 percent report changes in the governance structures of their hospitals, or clinical services, or both. Such changes include alterations in reporting relationships, a shift from hospital to health-system governance structures, a restructured faculty governance, mergers and joint ventures, privatization and creation of public authorities, and, in some cases, total restructuring of the clinical enterprise.

Health professions education. Many recent changes in the education arena are apparent, most notably, the downsizing of some programs and expansion of others, alterations in faculty reward systems, and more multiprofessional education. These changes continue a trend first noted in the 1992 survey.

For the majority of reporting institutions, funding for education had not suffered in the previous year. In fact, 45 percent of the respondents report an increase in state funding (58%, public; 21%, private institutions). In addition, 25 percent report increased educational support from their primary teaching hospitals (36% of freestanding academic health centers). On the other hand, although only 10 percent report decreases in state funding, 23 percent report decreased funds from their hospitals in the previous year. In our 1992 survey, decreases in state funding for education were reported by 59 institutions. It is important to note that the smaller number of institutions in the 1998 survey reporting decreases for the previous year may mask the fact that many had already seen cuts before then.

Table 4.
SOURCES OF FUNDS FOR EDUCATION, BY PERCENT

School	State	Tuition	Clinical Revenues	Other
Allied Health	47	36	8	14
Dentistry	50	23	16	13
Medicine	29	20	33	30
Nursing	54	38	10	17
Pharmacy	49	25	12	16
Public Health	36	45	8	30
Other	40	24	3	28

- Table 4 shows the average percentage of funds from various sources reported for education in the health professions schools. Predictably, medical schools are most dependent on clinical revenues (33%) and the least dependent on state funds (29%) and tuition (20%). Schools of allied health, dentistry, nursing, and pharmacy receive close to half their funding from the state, and clinical revenues account for 10 percent or less of the funding for schools of allied health, nursing, and public health.

- There is evidence of increased multiprofession education and sharing of resources across the health professions schools. In terms of basic science education, 29 respondents (40%) report that each health professions school has its own departments, 44 (61%) report that medical school faculty teach students from other schools and programs (up from 32 in 1992), and 8 (11%) report that the basic sciences are organized across the academic health center in such a way that students from various professions learn together. In terms of other courses, 40 respondents (56%) report shared courses across the professional schools, including didactic courses such as ethics, as well as a few clinical rotations and clerkships.

- The downsizing trend in the medical schools, residency, and fellowship programs that was reported in the 1992 and 1994 surveys continues. This time, 13 institutions report cutting full-time faculty, 39 report cutting specialty residency programs, and 26 report cutting fellowship programs. Four institutions report cuts in medical-school class size.

- Although not a dramatic change, downsizing as well as closure, of other schools and programs—especially nursing and allied health—also continues. Among the respondents, 8 institutions report decreasing faculty, and 9 report decreasing class size in a variety of lower-level nursing and allied health programs; 14 report closing down one or more programs, typically a small allied health program. This trend was noted first in 1992 and again in 1994.

- Downsizing in some areas is sometimes accompanied by expansion in others, which also continues a trend first noted in our 1992 survey, and which appears to have peaked in 1994. Twenty respondents, especially those in public institutions, report increases in upper-level nursing programs, mostly nurse practitioner and other advanced nurse clinician programs. In 1994, 52 reported such expansion! Many also have reported increases in physician assistant programs (18 in this survey, 26 in 1994) and such allied health programs as physical therapy, occupational therapy, and registered technologists (17 in this survey, 36 in 1994).

- Dramatic expansion of community-based educational sites continues. Thus, 53 institutions in this survey and 61 in 1994 have reported augmenting these sites in the previous year. Somewhat surprisingly, about two-thirds report that they have enough ambulatory sites for medical and other health professions students.

- There is substantial evidence that, after many years of discussion and considerable pressure for increased public accountability, faculty reward systems are changing. In 1992, 26 percent of the respondents reported that the tenure system was under review. In 1998, 22 percent report that the system had been changed in the previous year. Most of the changes included post-tenure reviews and faculty compensation changes. A total of 34 respondents (47%) said they have post-tenure review; of these, 8 institutions, all public and all university-based, report that post-tenure reviews had been state mandated. In addition, 19 report changes in faculty compensation systems in the previous year. Moreover, large numbers of the respondents report changes in the reward system to foster education and teaching (36%), primary care (37%), and research of all kinds (basic research, 17%; clinical research, 14%; and health services research, 13%).

Research. Many academic health centers are actively seeking to enhance their research activities, manage their research enterprise more efficiently, and encourage entrepreneurial research programs. Almost three-quarters (53) of respondents report that their research enterprises are not self-sufficient. Of these, 28 report the amount that needs to be subsidized from other sources, but 25 (19 from public academic health centers) are unsure of the amount. For those reporting lack of self-sufficiency, the mean amount of the shortfall is $17 million, with a range of $600,000 to $50 million, thus highlighting the great variability in the size of academic health center research activities.

- More than half the respondents (55%) report having established new alliances, joint ventures, or partnerships, or all three, in the previous year in an effort to support the research enterprise. These included alliances with industry, hospitals, and hospital systems; partnerships with other universities; and creating, or partnering with, research institutes. In addition, 32 institutions report that they had established new centers of excellence in the previous two years.

- We asked about the locus of decision making concerning the allocation of financial support, capital equipment, and space for research. It appears that within the same institution, some decisions are made by departments, some by individual schools, and some are centralized. Unfortunately, because of the way we worded the question, respondents' answers were not as informative as they could have been. Thus, we do not know what kinds of decisions are made at which level.

- Clearly, academic health centers are encouraging and managing entrepreneurial research activities. Eighty percent have technology transfer offices, and 75 percent have policies that give researchers financial incentives to engage in entrepreneurial activities, including distribution of a substantial proportion of the royalties. On average, the respondents report that 40 percent of the academic health centers give royalties to the investigator, 25 percent give to the department, 31 percent give to the investigator's school, and 28 percent give to other entities. (Not all institutions give to all categories.) The amount of royalties paid to the academic health center in the previous year is another measure of research intensity and of the variation among institutions. The mean amount reported was $3.7 million with a range of $0 to $60 million.

Clinical services. There is continuing evidence of trends seen in the 1992 and 1994 surveys: greater consolidation of the clinical enterprise, steps taken to improve efficiency, and development of linkages with other service providers and insurers as managed care continues to exert financial pressures on academic health centers and heightens competition in local marketplaces.

- More than half the respondents (38 institutions, or 53%) report that their academic health center has a single, comprehensive, multispecialty group practice. Another 15 institutions are actively working to implement a single practice plan, and 12 are in the conceptual stage. Only six institutions are not doing anything to move in this direction, and one did not answer this question on the survey. When asked about some of the details of the single practice plan, only 24 respondents report having a single patient record and a single appointment system, suggesting that not all the major administrative and management functions have been fully integrated. In terms of billing and collection, 39 respondents report having a single system for the practice plan, but only 10 report that the practice plan and hospital billing and collection systems are integrated.

- Half of the respondents report that their practice plan or plans include health professionals other than physicians. The most commonly mentioned were nurses, dentists, psychologists and social workers, and some allied health professionals.

- Although 65 percent of the institutions report that the practice plan has a single governance structure, only about one-quarter of those who own their own hospital report a single governance structure for both the hospital and practice plan.

- Finally, with regard to reporting relationships in the practice plan, one-third indicate that the head of the practice plan reports to the head of the academic health center, one-third to the dean of medicine, and one-third to a variety of other people. The academic health center leader and dean of medicine typically sit on the governing board of the practice plan along with departmental representatives and other administrators and faculty.

- In terms of patients admitted to the primary teaching hospital, approximately 25 percent are Medicare, 25 percent are Medicaid, and 22 percent are uninsured patients, according to the respondents. The mean amount of uncompensated care provided in the primary teaching hospital was $44 million (range $0 to $350 million), which is up from the 1992 survey when the mean reported was $29 million and the range was $10,000 to $272 million. Clearly the teaching hospitals are continuing, and perhaps even expanding, their service to the underserved in their communities.

- Ten respondents report that the status or ownership of their primary teaching hospital had changed in the previous year. Such changes include mergers with and acquisitions by both nonprofit and for-profit hospitals and health systems, forming a new entity with a nonprofit hospital to control clinical service management, and becoming a state or public authority. Hospital ownership today is not always as clear-cut as it used to be since, in some cases, universities share ownership and governance with other entities.

- Reports of downsizing the number of hospital beds and nursing and other staff continues a trend noticed in 1994. In 1998, 28 respondents report downsizing the number of active beds in their primary teaching hospital as compared with 32 in 1994; 33 report cutting nursing staff and 35 report cutting other hospital staff as compared with 43 and 47, respectively in 1994.

- Thirty percent (22 institutions) report having a university-owned HMO, and 22 percent (16 institutions) report having a university-owned insurance product, with another 8 institutions planning to develop such a product in the next year.

- Linkages with numerous other providers continue to proliferate and strengthen since we asked about it in 1994. As seen in table 5, most

Table 5.
ACADEMIC HEALTH CENTER LINKAGES WITH OTHER PROVIDERS

Type of linkage	Providers				
	Other hospitals	Community based physicians	Community health centers	Entities bringing substantial number of covered lives	Academic health centers in same city, state, or region
Bought	9	22	2	2	0
Merged with	8	1	0	1	0
Formed partnership with	13	20	5	12	8
Affiliated with	23	26	16	5	6
Contracted with	47	29	24	31	5
Held discussions with	33	27	12	26	19

respondents report partnerships, affiliations, and contracts with other hospitals, community-based physicians, and community health centers, as well as some strong connections to other academic health centers.

- Most academic health centers are part of a network or health system composed of an interrelated group of providers, including hospitals, physicians, and other clinical sites that have contractual agreements to deliver specific services. About 43 percent report being part of a network for all clinical services and another 33 percent report being part of a network for some clinical services.

- Finally, high proportions of the respondents report that their academic health centers have contractual agreements with new clinical partners providing support not only for undergraduate medical education (42%) and graduate medical education (46%), but also for other health professions education (25%), indigent care (18%), and research (22%). Interestingly, such support is somewhat more common among private institutions for medical education, indigent care, and research; among public institutions, it is higher for graduate medical education.

CONCLUSION

Change is evident in all mission areas of academic health centers. Perhaps the threat of managed care in and of itself has been enough to provoke significant institutional change. Restructuring, changes in rewards and incentives, consolidation of practice plans, and new partnerships for research and clinical services are especially noteworthy. Greater institutional flexibility, clinical efficiency, and selective downsizing and expansions are widespread and seem much less dependent on market stage than anticipated. What has not changed significantly is the role of the academic health center's chief executive officer, which continues to be strong and to span all mission areas. What a survey like this cannot show are the interesting details of particular institutional strategies that appear in the site visit report and case studies elsewhere in this volume.

CHAPTER 3

SITE VISIT REPORT

Kaludis Consulting Group

TO IDENTIFY SOME INNOVATIVE ADAPTATIONS TO the changing health care environment as well as some models for success the Kaludis Consulting Group visited the University of Cincinnati Medical Center, University of Colorado Health Sciences Center, University of Massachusetts Medical Center, and Baylor College of Medicine. The four academic health centers were selected because they reflected geographic and structural diversity and also had embarked on interesting approaches to change. During the visits, the study teams met one-on-one or in small groups with senior executives, selected department chairs and center or institute directors, representatives of clinical partners, and, where appropriate, university officials.

The two-day visits were an opportunity (1) to complement self-reporting (e.g., questionnaire completed by each center for the Association of Academic Health Centers) and (2) discuss challenges, issues, and transformational change. The conceptual framework was the impact of the changing clinical environment on education and research programs.

A summary of the institutional and health care market dynamics taking place at these institutions appears in table 1 and focuses on the innovations and strategies for success identified during those visits. In each visit, the clinical agenda tended to dominate the conversations. This situation is not surprising given that clinical services are so critical to the educational and economic priorities of academic health centers and that the institutions visited are still dealing with transformations in their markets for clinical services. The reality is that the clin-

Table 1.
INSTITUTIONAL CHARACTERISTICS AND HEALTH CARE MARKET DYNAMICS

	University of Cincinnati Medical Center	University of Colorado Health Sciences Center	University of Massachusetts Medical Center	Baylor College of Medicine
Location	Midwest	West	Northeast	Southwest
Control	Public	Public	Public	Private
Institutional status	Collocated with university	Academic health center campus, multicampus university	Academic health center campus, multicampus university	Standalone
Governance	State Board of Regents; most responsibilities delegated to 9-member, governor-appointed Board of Trustees	9-member publicly elected Board of Regents	19-member university system Board of Trustees (17 appointed by governor)	44-member self-perpetuating Board of Trustees
Academic programs	Medicine, nursing & center for health-related programs, pharmacy	Medicine, nursing, dentistry, pharmacy, graduate biomedical sciences	Medicine, nursing, graduate biomedical sciences	Medicine with allied health & graduate biomedical science components
Hospital status	Privatized	Public authority corporation	Owned hospital	No owned hospital
Academic health CEO	Senior vice president/ Provost, health affairs	Chancellor	Chancellor/Dean	President
Reporting relationship	University president	University system president	University system president	Board of Trustees
Operating budget (excluding clinical facilities)	$340 million	$341 million	$182 million	$549 million
NIH funding	45th in FY96: $37.6 million (30th when $26m from Children's Hospital Medical Center is counted)	22nd in FY96: $80.1 million	43rd in FY96: $43.4 million	17th in FY96: $89.1 million

	University of Cincinnati Medical Center	University of Colorado Health Sciences Center	University of Massachusetts Medical Center	Baylor College of Medicine
Students	2,883	2,229	435	1,174
Full-time faculty	969	2,042	721	1,455
Residents/Fellows	480	780	450	1,069
Managed care market	Stage IV	Stage III	Stage III	Early stage III
Status of Medicaid managed care	Mandate for statewide managed care by 2002; Hamilton County currently 50% mandated	About 30% recipients voluntarily enrolled in either HMO or PPO programs; legislation mandating at least 75% enrollment within 3 years	HMO or PPO option; approximately 30% recipients in capitated HMOs, 70% in PPO	Capitated Medicaid began 12/1/97
Clinical delivery system	Created new entity through virtual merger and hospital privatization	Separated hospital as public authority corporation; created virtual network with other hospitals	Formed through asset merger	Maintained teaching affiliations; building network with the Methodist Hospital
Market consolidation	3 clinical networks: TriHealth, Mercy System, Hospital Alliance of Greater Cincinnati	3 clinical networks: HealthCare Colorado; Centura; Columbia HCA/ Health One	5 clinical networks: Partners Health Care; Care Group; Tenet Corporation; LaheyHitchcock Health Care; Caritas Christi Health System	4 clinical networks: PhyCor/Med Partners; Memorial/ Sisters of Charity/ Hermann Hospital System; The Methodist Hospital/ MethodistCare; Texas Children's Hospital/Texas

The site visit discussions follow. For each institution, the overview identifies major initiatives that have had a significant effect on how each academic health center has moved out to meet and select its future. It flows from the study team's interpretation of the views and materials the center presented to the team. The discussion on innovations and strategies for success is anecdotal and not meant to be an exhaustive inventory of what is happening on campus.

BAYLOR COLLEGE OF MEDICINE

BAYLOR COLLEGE OF MEDICINE (BCM) IS A PRIVATE medical school located in the heart of Houston's Texas Medical Center. With graduate programs in the biomedical sciences, undergraduate degree programs in allied health, and a network of clinical teaching and practice affiliations that includes the Methodist Hospital, Texas Children's Hospital, the U.S. Department of Veteran's Affairs Medical Center, and the Harris County Hospital District, BCM is an academic health center.

The institution was founded in Dallas in 1900 and was affiliated with Baylor University from 1903 until 1969, when it became independent. The college moved to Houston in 1943 to become the educational cornerstone of the new Texas Medical Center. During the past half century, BCM has enjoyed unprecedented local political and financial support.

Historically blessed with strong leadership, BCM has never gone outside for its president, and the retiring presidents are made use of on a continuing basis, apparently without intruding on the independence of the new leader. In addition, a tradition of strong community and state support for Baylor has evolved over the years, in part, because of the prudent selection of major efforts to serve the public interest in creative and innovative ways over and above the traditional functions of an academic health center. Finally, because Baylor has never owned or operated any of its seven major affiliated hospitals, it has spent relatively little effort worrying about the changing health care delivery market. Houston became a competitive market relatively late in the game and, therefore, the BCM faculty has had more time than other academic health centers to prepare for the rigors of a more tightly managed market. Furthermore, the faculty has been able to push for national leadership in information technology, technology transfer, and educational entrepreneurship.

Circumstances have molded BCM into an institution that sustains its academic values even while being heavily leveraged. Because of its location in the Texas Medical Center, it has long had access to large-scale clinical operations without being beholden to one large clinical entity. Long-term relationships—with several private hospitals of the Medical Center, the Harris County Hospital District, and the Houston Veteran's Affairs Medical Center—as well as the state appropriation for undergraduate medical education, have placed BCM at the center of a network. BCM has not been marginalized by these network relationships, but has been able to stay close to the core of each of these universes. From its inception, BCM had to learn to move and act as a single entity in order to keep its head above water.

BCM has also built strong ties to philanthropic sources early and created a donor base that is one of its strongest financial assets. To this end, the institution has attracted and continues to attract high-quality people to its board of directors.

The college's executive leadership, moreover, has created considerable strategic space for the institution through national and international leadership in health care and research. Also, the image of the BCM president as master teacher and master physician has continued with each incumbent. For these reasons, BCM has been able to retain its capstone role in clinical medicine and research in Houston and beyond. It recognizes, however, that retention of the capstone role will require more focused planning and capital investment and increased flexibility and institutional responsiveness. Like its academic health center siblings, BCM is moving to a stronger mission management approach with particular attention to how it can use its franchise more effectively in the international clinical and medical education spheres.

UNIQUE STRENGTHS

Baylor College of Medicine is somewhat unique among academic health centers because it is a private, stand-alone medical school that has never owned a hospital. In addition, major portions of the academic enterprise operate on the margins of other educational and clinical institutions, including Rice University, University of Houston, Texas Woman's University, and seven major public and private affiliated teaching hospitals. These partnerships allow BCM to play "bigger than it is," that is, to focus its resources on core activities.

Beginning with its relocation in 1943 to the new Texas Medical Center, which has developed into one of the world's leading health care institutions, BCM has experienced unprecedented growth. Its success is also due to the charismatic leadership of BCM Chancellor Emeritus Dr. Michael E. DeBakey who captured the imagination of Houston. Early on, DeBakey helped BCM to build strong political, social, and economic alliances and establish deep roots among the city's power brokers.

Today, BCM ranks ninth among academic health centers in total extra-mural funding. And, despite being a private institution, it receives extraordinary support from the state, which allocated $30 million to BCM for 1996/97, con-tinuing a public-private partnership launched with the More Doctors for Texas initiative in the early 1970s. This level of public funding is greater than that received by some public academic health centers.

GOALS

BCM's aspirations are ambitious: to become one of the top five academic health centers by 2005 and to capture one-third of the clinical market share in the greater Houston area. The expectation in virtually every quarter is that these goals will be met. Baylor's private clinical partners are very strong financially, with combined reserves in excess of $4 billion, providing an almost unparalleled source of venture capital for faculty recruitment, clinical outreach, and research development.

The strategy for reaching the top five has three prongs:

- Invest in current strengths (maintain current top five programs).
- Anticipate science to capitalize on intellectual and resource opportunities.
- Identify and remedy intolerable weaknesses that would preempt the top five status if left unattended.

Capturing a 33 percent clinical market share is potentially a more elusive goal. Houston is a late Stage II–early Stage III managed care market, with little capitation, although capitated Medicaid has just been introduced. Because the Harris County Hospital District's hospitals and community health centers are integral elements of BCM's clinical education and service enterprise, the effects of Medicaid managed care on these institutions is of particular interest.

MERGER STRATEGY

The recent announcement of the Memorial Hospital System/Hermann Hospital merger marks a new stage of market consolidation. Prior to the merg-er, consolidation was focused primarily in the proprietary arena, where

Columbia/HCA and Tenet went about the business of building their networks, with seventeen and five hospitals, respectively. The Memorial/Hermann merger will give this new system about a 20 percent market share, just on the heels of Columbia/HCA's 21 percent. It also changes the dynamics among Texas Medical Center institutions, giving Memorial a presence there when Columbia/HCA has none, and giving Hermann access to Memorial's broad network, something its medical center competitors, Methodist Health Care System and St. Luke's Episcopal Hospital, lack. The new system will have combined revenues of more than $2 billion, 2,500 operating beds, and 11,000 employees, making it a formidable force and giving a boost to the medical school at the University-Houston Health Science Center for which Hermann is the major private, not-for-profit teaching hospital. This market realignment makes the success of Baylor's new initiatives to strengthen its financial linkages with both Methodist Health Care System and Texas Children's Hospital even more important.

One significant managerial characteristic of Baylor is an executive cadre composed of part-time doctors. This began with Dr. DeBakey, who operated almost every day of his presidency, and continues today as the president, vice presidents, deans, and associate deans continue to be active in teaching, research, and clinical service. This approach worked, and worked well, when environmental and institutional circumstances did not require a lot of managerial attention. As the management agenda becomes more complex, however, it remains to be seen whether this model can continue to provide the necessary leadership.

ACCOMPLISHMENTS

Meanwhile, a number of innovations have been put in place. Among the steps Baylor has taken are the following:

- Strengthened its partnership with Methodist Hospital by creating Baylor Methodist Primary Care Specialists as a 501(a) corporation with the goal of hiring 240 family medicine and general internal medicine physicians within five years. A similar initiative was launched with Texas Children's Hospital, another 501(a) corporation, to purchase the practices of 109 primary care pediatricians in five years. In two and a half years, the corporation already employed 146 pediatricians with investment recovered and positive cash flow.

- Created Affiliated Medical Services in partnership with the school of medicine at the University of Texas–Houston Health Science Center. The new entity is a 501(a) corporation that allows for a single point of integration (interface/negotiation) for contracting with the Harris County Hospital District for services at its public hospitals and health centers.

- Introduced an educational assessment by every learner at every encounter (rotation, lecture, ward attending, small groups/labs).

- Changed tenure policy to narrow the scope of tenure to be tenure of title, not salary or space; this took away the economic value of tenure. The tenure decision timeline is now nine years with the opportunity to shift to the nontenure track, compared to the norm of seven years, up or out.

- Enhanced interdisciplinary/multiprofessional education, research, and academic services, including (1) a 24-credit-hour service (core) curriculum; (2) three interdisciplinary departments in the graduate school where faculty collaborate with faculty from Rice University and the University of Texas–Houston Health Science Center; (3) common basic science (anatomy, physiology, biochemistry, and most of pharmacology) instruction and integrated clinical training for MD, PA, and CNRA students; and (4) integrated orientation, convocation, and graduation across allied health, graduate, and medical student bodies.

- Established the Office of Outcomes Management to address a range of performance and productivity issues, including patient satisfaction, clinical efficiency, practice standards, payor/referring physician satisfaction, resource utilization, and preferred clinical pathways.

- Started to implement Baylor Metrics, a set of key performance measures for faculty and staff in all three mission areas—education, research, and clinical service—to guide allocation, recapture, and reallocation of resources.

- Organized clinical contract research through a contract research organization (CRO) with centralized support resources, a speedy institutional review board (IRB) process, and faculty alignment for rapid production.

- Established a major outsourcing relationship with ServiceMaster for broad support services (food service, housekeeping, grounds, information technology) to simplify management, integrate risk sharing, and establish strong incentives to increase customer satisfaction.

- Created its own satellite television channel, seeking to capitalize on technological distribution possibilities. "The Health Channel" delivers continuing education courses, news reports on medical breakthroughs, and other programs on a subscription basis, packaged with an entertainment product. A major distinguishing feature of the Baylor plan is that, unlike other experiments with televised medical education programming, this one allows subscribers to take continuing education courses via the channel without paying tuition. In addition to subscriber fees, the college expects to make money from the sale of video and multimedia products created from broadcast programs.

- Aggressively pursued clinical medicine opportunities in such far-flung locations as Russia, Peru, and Malaysia in response to a potentially growing excess clinical capacity resulting from increased managed care penetration in the Houston market.

STRATEGIES FOR SUCCESS

- Think big and have a can-do attitude! The history of the institution and the Texas Medical Center is filled with example after example of bold visions becoming reality. The ability to recognize and exploit opportunity is quintessentially Houstonian. "The Health Channel" and international medicine are just two examples.

- Pick your partners wisely. The financial capabilities of Baylor's private clinical partners provide an uncommon advantage.

- Capture the philanthropic high ground. When it was the only medical school in town, Baylor and M.D. Anderson Hospital (now the University of Texas M.D. Anderson Cancer Center) firmly established themselves as the philanthropy of choice among the rich and famous. Both institutions continue to reap substantial rewards, as evidenced by Baylor's successful $500 million capital campaign.

- Make internal appointments for leadership succession with continuing roles for former CEOs. In Baylor's experience, this kind of succession provides for smooth, short transitions and some measure of strategic continuity.
- Use an all-funds budgeting process to identify the economic realities of its core missions and allow for more informed investment decisions.

UNIVERSITY OF CINCINNATI MEDICAL CENTER

THE UNIVERSITY OF CINCINNATI (UC) AROSE OUT OF a confederation of the schools of medicine and law. It is classified as a Research I institution and relies on the research strength of the College of Medicine to maintain that designation. Since joining the state university system in 1979, UC has enjoyed strong political and financial support, particularly for capital construction. However, in recent years, general fund support from the state has been less than it has been for other institutions in the system, thereby pushing tuition rates up.

The University of Cincinnati Medical Center (UCMC) comprises the Colleges of Medicine, Nursing, Health, and Pharmacy and the Hoxworth Blood Center. It is affiliated with University Hospital, a member of the Health Alliance of Greater Cincinnati.

A leadership/environmental dyad was established. The new university president arrived and recruited an internationally known clinician-investigator to serve as the vice president for health affairs. Within a few years the tensions between a well-established departmental imperative and the need for collective or corporate action were elevated to a test of university resolve. Vice presidential, presidential, and trustee commitment to establish the administrative and leadership capacity necessary to act collectively and thereby accomplish change was clearly demonstrated. Thus, the stage was set for more dramatic action with full departmental support.

After moving the faculty clinical practice toward a comprehensive group practice, enhancing the management and profitability of the hospital, and developing a health maintenance organization, the institution was positioned to help create a large hospital system in which it would participate.

UCMC is a prime example of how a new framework for an academic health center can be created and how strong support from the parent university can help an academic health center.

Moving swiftly in anticipation of health care market competition, UCMC accomplished the following over a 23-month period:

1. Privatized its own hospital.
2. Developed new operating agreements with previous competitor hospitals leading to the creation of a major network of not-for-profit groups, the Health Alliance of Greater Cincinnati (HAGC).
3. Anticipated the need for a new physician model by designing and implementing the Alliance Physicians Service (APS), a physician contracting and services group that serves both faculty physicians and private physicians.
4. Won a public referendum for continuation of a tax levy that supports indigent care at the medical center, a vote held periodically, thus requiring that the academic health center continue to be grounded in the values and needs of its community.
5. Resolved support-service and cost-allocation issues with UC resulting from the privatization of the hospital.
6. Began an internal reassessment and restructuring to fit the context that its leadership had created.
7. Through Alliance Partners (the Alliance), closed one of its facilities and transferred part of that facility's franchise to another location, thereby passing its first major test.

The import of the UC approach is that UCMC, with the support of the university, recognized and acted on strategic health care market issues before it was too late, including altering its own internal clinical and educational corporate structure. In so doing, UC pitted the issue of the long-term viability of the medical center against short-term and special interests. The longer-term perspective prevailed.

The university's board and its president were mobilized and out front in advocating for the monumental changes that consequently took place, unequivocally supporting the medical center and its leadership in its bold steps. Labor and other interest groups pressed hard against hospital privatization. Nevertheless, the clear message was that the public expected UC to operate on a businesslike basis, but with significant local tax support. The local corporate community was surprised and pleased that UC had the ability to make these moves, generating a new level of respect for a university and medical center able to rise up and represent institutionwide interests.

UCMC also chose to draw new strategic boundaries in both the clinical facility and physician participation sectors. The expectation was that the medical center would thereby be able to respond more effectively to carrying out a set of real relationships than they would if they operated under some manufactured sense of the future. Thus, the ethos of planning and management at the medical center has been fundamentally altered, although it is as yet too early to know the full impact.

CREATING AN INTEGRATED
HEALTH SYSTEM

Early in his tenure, the vice president for health affairs, recognizing that resource constraints would intensify over the years, set in motion a long-term strategy to align resources with priorities, strengthen the research enterprise, and develop an integrated system for health care delivery. By 1995, a comprehensive integrated health system had been established through the formation of three linked corporations, as follows:

1. HAGC, a virtual (nonasset) merger of University Hospital and Christ Hospital (later expanded with the addition of St. Luke's and Jewish Hospitals), with common governance and management, a single strategic plan, and shared bottom line.

2. APS created to link members of the faculty group practice with community practitioners (except for primary care physicians who are part of one of HAGC's four divisions: Hospitals, Rehabilitation/Home Health, Primary Care, and Education and Research).

3. The Alliance, a voluntary management services organization (MSO) capitalized by the other two corporations.

The structures of the new corporations preserve a governance role for the

UCMC leadership and set the stage for the creation of a structure to ensure long-term financial support for the academic mission.

In an additional step, University Hospital was privatized to give it greater flexibility in a rapidly changing market, and to insulate the university from the risk of the health care delivery business while supporting education and research. With privatization, University Hospital's senior executive officer is accountable to the Alliance CEO, not to the vice president for health affairs. University Hospital accountability to the UCMC for continued orientation to the academic mission is uncertain. Ensuring the future development of the Alliance as an integrated health care delivery system in ways that meet educational needs (quality, quantity, mix of patients) is an ongoing priority and challenge for the UCMC leadership.

Prior to formation of the Alliance, Cincinnati had witnessed rapid consolidation of health care plans and UC concluded that a merger was essential to sustain the long-term viability of University Hospital. In the pre-Alliance market, the UCMC clinical faculty had access to significant numbers of covered lives through various health plans, but University Hospital was included for only 10 percent of the covered lives in the city. Hospital alignments now appear to be in place; there are no proprietary hospital companies in the market, and only one community hospital seems vulnerable to closure in the near future.

Continuing clinical success is marked by increased market share for the Alliance, University Hospital, and UC Medical Asociates (UCMA), a faculty group practice. University Hospital's patient volume is increasing in a declining patient-volume market. Annual UCMA practice volume increases are averaging between 7 percent and 10 percent. Primary care practices continue to grow, with more than 180 physicians now practicing at forty-eight sites throughout the tristate area.

The creation of the Alliance and privatization of University Hospital were accomplished through the visionary leadership of a small number of people in a climate of trust. Goodwill and shared vision were essential. As in any partnership, the departure of a key leader has the potential to destabilize relationships. Therefore, efforts are underway to institutionalize a decision-making framework for support of the academic mission.

A proposed Division of Education and Research, to be led by the dean of the College of Medicine, is envisioned as the umbrella for residency training programs, medical student education in hospitals, continuing medical education, institutional review board, clinical research, and libraries and informatics. This division is to be funded by 1.5 percent of HAGC gross revenues and up to 1.5 percent of gross revenues on new managed care contracts of Alliance Partners. Use of these funds will be proposed by the medical center and approved by HAGC. The structure is about to be put in place and the funding and resource allocation mechanism to be activated. Neither structure nor accountability, however, will address the problem of melding disparate cultures (academic, community, and hospital) within HAGC.

RESULTS

UCMC has successfully completed the complex challenge of gaining approval of privatization while, at the same time, winning renewal of the tax levy to support indigent care at University Hospital. Although much progress has been made since the Alliance was created, the difficult but essential work of service-line consolidation and right-sizing the workforce is only beginning. The impact of these changes on education and clinical research is yet to be understood.

The risks are considerable: University Hospital could move away from the academic model as the economics of managed care become the bottom line. The educational network could be at risk as affiliated institutions terminate clerkships essential for accreditation. The clinical supervision of students could be linked to payments from the college of medicine, diverting resources from research support. In addition, teaching faculty could reduce or even cease their involvement in education under the competitive pressures of managed care. Faculty are concerned about the economics of managed care (e.g., the need to increase the workload significantly to maintain the financial status quo) and its effect on their ability to pay attention to education (and, to a lesser degree, research).

Meanwhile, a number of innovations are in place, as follows:

- The Institute for Health Policy and Health Services Research now has a Center for Clinical Effectiveness as its largest unit, with emphasis on clinical outcomes, practice evaluation, and dissemination of information about clinical effectiveness.

- Funds from the state technology initiative are being matched with institutional resources to finance a fiber optic upgrade for the UC campus communications network.

- The UCMC has founded a biomedical incubator facility, Bio/Start, with institutional funds, private gifts, and space leased from the Alliance. Bio/Start provides space, legal, and marketing support to fledgling biotechnology companies.

- A faculty-group practice, UCMA has sold assets (primary care, satellite buildings, and patient information system) to Alliance Partners, which has recognized the economies of scale in centralized business systems and offered services to non-UCMA users, reducing the aggregate UCMA overhead by more than $1.5 million per year.

- The Department of Psychiatry became an early innovator in the shift from clinical service delivery care to a blend of clinical service delivery and behavioral medicine management by entering into contracts with state agencies to manage mental health service delivery.

- The medical center, HAGC, and the College of Business have created a successful physician leadership course (32 weeks; 128 contact hours) to address the challenge of blending the complex cultures of the health care community and academic health center.

STRATEGIES FOR SUCCESS

- Make strategic decisions quickly and communicate, communicate, communicate the who, what, where, when, why, and how at every step along the way. Build communication around answers to questions of individual self-interest. (How will change affect me or my job?)

- Focus resources on research in areas where UC could realistically be a national leader with the goal of moving into the top 20 among medical schools for NIH funding.

- Increase the quality of students in all programs.

- Capitalize on the opportunity to establish an operating model between UCMC and HAGC comparable to that between UCMC and Children's Hospital in which support for the 225-member pediatric faculty is provided by Children's Hospital and the Children's Hospital

Research Foundation.

- Position UCMC as a strong player in the strongest comprehensive integrated health care delivery system in Cincinnati. Create an Education and Research Division within the Alliance to secure long-term financial support for the academic mission.

- Position the faculty group practice to exert more influence on the health care system through their dominant role in APS.

- Allow market forces and competition among systems to determine the appropriate number of hospitals, beds, and specialists for the metropolitan area.

- Optimize the use of information technology. An intense drive by HAGC and UCMC to establish a comprehensive, integrated information system now links forty-eight delivery sites and the five hospitals with all elements of the medical center.

- Maintain the position of Children's Hospital and University Hospital as the sole providers of pediatric care for the indigent, and the predominant provider of pediatric care for the tristate area.

THE UNIVERSITY OF COLORADO HEALTH SCIENCES CENTER

T HE UNIVERSITY OF COLORADO HEALTH SCIENCES Center (UCHSC), one of four campuses of the University of Colorado, is made up of the Schools of Medicine, Nursing, Pharmacy, and Dentistry, a graduate school, a variety of research and patient care institutes, and two teaching hospitals. It has an externally oriented, highly leveraged economy (only 9% of revenues come from state appropriations, tuition, and fees), employing an all-funds budget that allows for more informed resource allocation decisions.

A NEW ORDER

The Kaludis Consulting Group view is that a long history of leadership struggles between powerful departmental chairs, chairs and deans, and deans and vice presidents, coupled with indifferent leadership at the university level, set the stage for action by a new, politically savvy university president and a group of trustees tired of useless internal struggling.

Their decision was to seek a strong vice president for the health center who, in turn, joined forces with a new cadre of deans and a leading hospital administrator to move the institution forward. The most powerful chairs also have come aboard.

The first major objective was freeing the hospital from some unnecessary shackles of bureaucracy and developing and implementing a new strategic plan aimed at cutting costs and increasing clinical market share. Having progressed further than many other academic health centers in this regard, Colorado has turned toward the development of innovative educational programs and the evolution of an already significant research enterprise.

Hemmed in by its neighborhood, the institution also has embarked on a dramatic transformational venture to relocate the entire campus to a large site a number of miles away, the former Fitzsimons Army Hospital site, over the next several years and even decades. The move represents much more than a real estate deal. Positioning the University of Colorado Health Sciences Center as a local, state, regional, national, and international health education, research, and service organization is the strategic aim of the move. The new location anticipates the growth of the metropolitan Denver area and places the Health Sciences Center at major air and automobile transportation hubs.

The Fitzsimons strategy has created a unique management challenge by requiring a balancing of investment and initiative between the current and new sites, suggesting the need for a three-pronged approach: planning and management for the current model; planning and management for the new model; and planning and management for the two together.

The political fallout from the proposed move continues, but, if the Fitzsimons initiative is to succeed, stable, strong executive leadership will be required. Unfortunately, a leadership change recently occurred at the health center with the resignation of the chancellor.

THE HEALTH SCIENCES CENTER

All four of the health professions schools have a strong research focus, and the Schools of Nursing and Pharmacy rank among the top ten in extramural research funding for their disciplines. Across UCHSC, NIH extramural funding has increased by about 10 percent a year above the national average, and the current leadership emphasizes cross-disciplinary collaboration as a key research strategy for the future. The research enterprise is highly leveraged and, potentially, at risk. The economic hydraulics of research depend, in part, on the clinical enterprise. Funds from clinical practice flow to the Academic Enrichment Fund, which allocates funds to basic science departments to support research. As managed care squeezes margins and shifts market share, the amount of monies flowing into the Academic Enrichment Fund could decrease.

Clinical research may be at even greater risk. If clinical services are eliminated or shuffled as a result of managed care, the clinical research milieu changes. Some faculty have indicated that the cost of a research-friendly clinical environment may be higher than that of an education-friendly one. Historically, public support for higher education has not been vigorous in Colorado despite the high mean educational attainment level of its citizens. UCHSC ranks below the average for Colorado universities in receipt of total state general funds and in receipt of general fund dollars per full-time student. The state general fund appropriation to UCHSC remained essentially flat from 1989/90 through 1994/95. After adjusting 1989/90 for the final year of indigent care funds for University Hospital, the annual increases averaged less than $1 million. In 1995/96, the state general fund appropriation took a modest upswing of $3.2 million, to $59.6 million.

In 1989, the Colorado legislature gave the board of regents of the University of Colorado authority to reorganize the hospital, and in 1991, University Hospital was converted from a state agency to a public authority, governed by a nine-member board and linked to UCHSC's academic mission. The Colorado Psychiatric Hospital remains an entity within UCHSC and provides services in five locations. Pediatric research and clinical programs are located in the affiliated Denver Children's Hospital. University Hospital, a public authority corporation, is nimble and flexible compared to the other components of the academic health center, which are encumbered by state human resource and procurement policies and procedures.

Three major health systems have emerged in Colorado in the last decade: Columbia HCA/Health One, Centura, and the UCHSC system alliance,

HealthCare Colorado. The UCHSC alliance comprises University Hospital, Denver Health Medical Center, Exempla Hospitals (St. Joseph's and Lutheran), Poudre Valley–Ft. Collins, Longmont United, Boulder Community, Colorado Springs Memorial, Park View Pueblo, and San Luis Valley Regional Medical Center.

Columbia HCA/Health One spent $500 million to try to buy a 30 percent market share. It was unsuccessful in its efforts to purchase Children's Hospital, however, and, therefore, plans to develop its own comprehensive pediatric services at Presbyterian St. Luke's Hospital. This could be a threat to Children's Hospital (and, potentially, pediatric education and research) if it were to draw away patients. Through HealthCare Colorado, University Hospital has enhanced its relationships with community hospitals and community health centers, building on the partnerships created in Colorado Access, the largest Medicaid managed care organization in the state.

As an example of building market alignment pressures, Children's Hospital was forced to withdraw from its equity position in HealthCare Colorado by Centura, whose referrals have historically accounted for 30 to 40 percent of Children's business.

UCHSC faces its own dilemma. As the market alignment drives it toward participation in a single health system, UCHSC finds that it continues to need the resources of multiple systems (including clinical competitors) to support its medical student and resident education programs adequately. And the squeeze on education is only likely to intensify as the managed care market matures.

UCHSC has major requirements for research and instructional space that cannot be met at the current site because of expansion limitations imposed by the city in what has been a sometimes tense town-gown struggle (including threats of lawsuits by the mayor of Denver) and because of building limitations imposed by the board of regents. The inability to build on university land west of Colorado Boulevard prompted a search for a second campus. As a result of the Federal Base Relocation and Closure (BRAC) Act of 1988, the 350-acre Fitzsimons Army Medical Center became available. In 1996, the board approved the relocation of the campus to Fitzsimons over a fifty-year period. However, the UCHSC believes it needs a five- to ten-year development period to plan and execute the move. The estimated price tag is $1 billion.

The impending move has generated a lot of controversy, raising such questions as: Does UCHSC have the human and infrastructure resources to maintain two campuses? Is a fifty-year transition period (two generations) too long? How will geographic separation from clinical affiliates affect educational programs?

A number of innovations are in place as follows:

- Separation of University Hospital into a public authority has provided badly needed flexibility in terms of personnel, purchasing, and decision-making, while preserving a link to the academic health center mission.

- The new leadership structure has included a developing role for physicians in hospital governance and management. In place of historic side deals between clinical department chairs and hospital administration, the Clinical Chairs Management Committee reviews and sets priorities for all requests for hospital funds, chairs don't seek funding without committee approval, and the dean is notified by the hospital director of all funding to departments.

- The School of Dentistry requires that all students spend a full academic year in service to underserved populations. Under supervision in both urban and rural clinic sites, students were expected to provide about $1.5 million worth of care to the underprivileged in 1996/97. The school was founded with a mission to provide dental professionals for rural, underserved communities in the state. As positions in rural communities were filled, the mission focus has shifted to underserved populations in both urban and rural locales.

- UCHSC sought permission from the Colorado Commission on Higher Education to initiate a new doctoral program in clinical science in 1997. This would be a minimum four-year curriculum designed to prepare physicians, graduate students, and other health professionals for careers in health services research or clinical investigations.

- The chancellor created an Office for Interdisciplinary Education and charged the four health professions deans with developing new cross-disciplinary curricula. The dean of dentistry took responsibility for developing the first offering—a course on professionalism for all students in doctoral programs in the health professions.

- The School of Medicine has implemented a new, three-pronged, market-driven compensation model, called BSI (base, supplement, and incentive), for clinical and basic science faculty.

- Tenure has been disassociated from promotion, with discontinuation of the up-or-out provision. Further, the financial value of tenure has been set at base salary, with base salary being small and fixed by rank across all medical disciplines.

- The School of Dentistry has developed a state-of-the-art clinic by soliciting equipment donations from major dental equipment manufacturers, creating a unique continuing education opportunity for alumni and other practitioners around the state to test leading-edge dental technology and provide useful feedback to the manufacturers.

- In fall 1997, UCHSC unified the graduate programs in biomedical sciences with a common entry system and common core curriculum, and later moved to a common graduate degree. Enrollment limits have not been set, but the intent is to cap the program.

- The School of Medicine has introduced an Individual Practice Agreement (IPA) that controls new faculty access to contracted patients as a means of influencing faculty behavior and preempting competition by introducing limitations on a physician's ability to compete in the geographic area if they leave the faculty.

- UCHSC has established the University Scientist Program (USP) to pool consulting income (operational in 1998). The funds will be used for faculty salary support and to provide incentives to faculty for developing collaborations with industry. Consulting income generated under the USP will also be subject to a 10 percent tax by the School of Medicine Academic Enrichment Fund, which will contribute the money to the enhancement of academic programs. Specific distribution decisions will be governed by departmental incentive plans, which will be developed and adopted by a majority vote of the respective department faculty.

STRATEGIES FOR SUCCESS

- Have a big, bold vision (Fitzsimons) and sell it aggressively. The more ambitious the vision, the easier it is to create the bandwagon effect because people can usually find some aspect of it that addresses their self-interest.

- Position University Hospital to compete effectively in the managed care marketplace.

- Develop community alliances while continuing to create a niche for UCHSC as the leading regional provider of quaternary care.

- Develop University Physicians, Inc. (faculty practice) as a single, non-profit corporation charged with management of the clinical practice, maintenance of physician provider networks, development of service contracts, and management of the group practice finances.

- Empower physicians while retaining linkage between the dean of medicine and the practice group.

- Relocate the health sciences center campus to Fitzsimons Army Medical Center to permit needed expansion in alignment with the shifting of metropolitan Denver's population and in proximity to potential biotechnology partners.

- Continue to build research excellence by fostering cross-disciplinary programs in basic research and enhancing clinical and translational research.

- Conduct excellent educational programs in the health professions with special focus on preparing graduates for the unique needs of the state and region.

- Maximize effective use of communications technologies and medical informatics to succeed with Fitzsimons strategy.

UNIVERSITY OF MASSACHUSETTS
MEDICAL CENTER

T
HE UNIVERSITY OF MASSACHUSETTS MEDICAL CENTER (UMMC), one of five campuses of the University of Massachusetts, includes schools of medicine and nursing, a graduate school of biomedical sciences, a variety of centers and institutes, and the UMass Health System. Located in central Massachusetts, the university was founded in 1962 (the first class was admitted in 1970), with the mission of educating health professionals for the state and providing care to the people of central and western Massachusetts.

The medical center's birth was met with a measure of skepticism by many, including legislators, pundits, and academic health professionals in eastern Massachusetts who felt it was being built in the wrong place at the wrong time. Subsequent legislative efforts to sink the institution, combined with the frontier-like culture of starting a new school in isolation from the Boston academic world, combined to forge an almost unequaled loyalty and commitment to and love for the institution by faculty and administrators. Out of its "newness" and isolation, a genuine sense of community was born at UMMC. The institution's nurturing culture is best exemplified by the current chancellor/dean, whose leadership skills have positioned the institution for even greater success.

Although younger than the majority of academic health centers, UMMC at age 35 has reached a level of institutional maturity and success that equals or exceeds many of the public and private medical schools created both before and after the 1960s. Despite declines in research productivity linked to the budget-cutting climate, UMMC's research enterprise has flourished over the last 23 years, and is currently ranked forty-third in National Institutes of Health (NIH) extramural funding. Furthermore, its growth rate in NIH funding for FY96 was the highest among the top fifty medical schools; UMMC ranked twelfth of all medical schools in total NIH funding growth.

The growth of a campus famous for having been declared dead on arrival is one of the top success stories among the twenty or so academic health centers that were created in the late sixties and early seventies. Partly because it was born in a hostile environment and partly because of hyperintense political and public scrutiny, the leaders of the departments and the faculty at large have always tended to be more team-oriented and institution-minded than those at other academic health centers. This team orientation has created a particular strategic niche for UMMC.

The academic health center is blessed with a leader who communicates exceedingly well with both internal and external constituents, and great progress has been made on many fronts. The leader has ensured that the political apparatus of the community and state feel included in the affairs of the institution and do not feel as though they are being held in abeyance by a distant or arrogant faculty. The university leadership is supportive and has fostered flexibility of action for the academic health center in many ways.

THE MERGER

UMMC assured its clinical survival by joining forces with its most powerful competitor, Memorial Health Care (MHC), in a new, merged system (UMass Memorial Health Care), in which control is shared jointly through a new board. The first two CEOs took turns serving as chair of the board. Government contracts for service, research, and teaching have tied the institution more fully to the interests and constituencies of the state. Mergers on the research front with the private, nonprofit Worcester Foundation, the proximity of a research park, and liaisons with state toxicology labs and pathology services all are contributing to the diversification of the academic health center's economic portfolio and educational milieu.

Internally, the administration has established centralized executive leadership for research, for education, and for clinical care. This has resulted in planning across departments as well as institution-wide sharing of resources in each of the three product lines, or mission areas. These developments have led to ongoing discussions about the changing roles of departmental chairs and about strategies for the sustenance of such leaders despite an altered portfolio.

From its inception, UMMC, out of necessity, learned to operate as one entity. The need to survive in a hostile environment galvanized this effort. As it matured, UMMC has become an example of an academic health center that developed a strong institutional medicine strategy, moving aggressively to get the state and its agencies to see it as a special and competent resource for providing health care services. More than many other academic health centers, the UMMC situation has been skewed toward an agenda for the whole, and its ethos is reflected in the consequences.

Central Massachusetts is currently a Stage III (consolidation) managed care marketplace with minimal capitation penetration (about 2.5%). However, penetration is expected to accelerate as the state shifts Medicaid emphasis from the modified fee-for-service Primary Care Clinician Program to the capitated health maintenance organization option. As in most markets, the introduction and growth of Medicaid capitation is expected to introduce changes in faculty practice and clinical service delivery that will have an impact on the educational programs.

The merger of UMMC and MHC will solidify the university's market dominance as the complementary strengths of each clinical enterprise come together synergistically. The educational programs will likely be affected by market realignment and consolidation because significant portions of the internal medicine and pediatric clerkships (as much as one-third and one-half, respectively) are provided by educational partners aligned with competing networks (e.g., St. Vincent/Fallon-Tenet). It is the changing clinical landscape that puts the educational enterprise at risk.

INNOVATIONS

Meanwhile, a number of innovations have been put in place, as follows:

- A financial arrangement for education and research support was negotiated up front as part of the merger agreement. Unlike many institutions where education and research interests are overshadowed by the clinical marketplace, the UMass/HMC agreement specifies the level of investment in education and research to be made by the clinical enterprise. Helping the negotiations was the fact that HMC's CEO is a professor of medicine and an active faculty member at UMMC who understands not only the complexities of the education and research enterprises, but also their competitive value to the clinical enterprise.

- A vice chancellor for education was appointed to act as an integrative force in curricula development, teaching effectiveness, education outcomes assessment, graduate medical education (GME) planning and evaluation, and clinical education network development.

- The role of the Educational Policy Committee (curriculum) was changed from being department bound to one that is institution bound, signaling a philosophical shift in the management of the institution. This set the stage for an integrated curriculum.

- In forming the new clinical network, UMMC established a single development office reporting to the chancellor/dean, allowing for more effective allocation and management of philanthropic resources, and eliminating the usual tension between academic and clinical organizations.

STRATEGIES FOR SUCCESS

1. *Understand the mission.* From the beginning, UMMC recognized that it was different from Harvard or Tufts and never tried to be something it wasn't.

2. *Stick with clinical strategy even if initial overtures are rebuffed.* Even though MHC initially rejected UMMC's overtures and the university was forced to pursue other options aggressively, the synergistic potential of a UMass/Memorial merger was in the end so strong that the follow-up overture was welcomed.

3. *Convert the organizational structure from departmentally focused to institutionally focused.* UMMC combined leadership positions into one, e.g., chancellor/dean, and superimposed a mission-focused organization (with single executives for education, research, and clinical service) on the departmental structure to create a matrix organization in which the role of the department chair is changing but not yet completely redefined. This gave the chancellor/dean the opportunity to recruit department chairs who understood the institutional context.

4. *Create a single point of authority to attack a decentralized, nonprimary care academic health center with chair fiefdoms and independent deals.* UMMC created the position of deputy chancellor for clinical affairs.

5. *Push institutional medicine opportunities through service agreements with state agencies.* UMMC, for example, signed agreements with the

Massachusetts Department of Mental Health, Department of Corrections, and Division of Medical Security.

6. *Set up competitive pools of resources for educational improvement.* UMMC has invested some $600,000 in a combination of salary supplements for course and clerkship directors and curriculum development funds. The latter are allocated by competitive request, with faculty submitting proposals for review by the vice chancellor for education and the chair of the educational policy committee.

7. *Develop a single, nonprofit corporation charged with management of the clinical practice, maintenance of physician-provider networks, development of service contracts, and financial management of the group practice.* UMMC created University Physicians, Inc., which empowered physicians while retaining linkage between the dean of medicine and the practice group.

8. *Benefit from relatively stable and economically productive faculty.* As a new institution, UMMC recruited young faculty with potential, and turnover has been extremely low. Faculty potential has translated into a growing research base, with minimal unfunded research.

9. *Reward research investigators and their academic departments with funds for research purposes based on the amount of indirect cost recovery.*

10. *Develop solid graduate biomedical science doctoral programs as the foundation on which to build nationally and internationally significant research programs.*

CHAPTER 4

DEVELOPMENT OF
THE NEW ROLE OF THE
CLINICAL CHAIR

Julien F. Biebuyck, MB, DPhil

> *Perhaps nowhere in the evolving academic medical center will the impact
> of change be more stressful and consequential than for the TRADITIONAL
> clinical academic chair, who I believe is an endangered species.*

David Korn (1996)

TWO YEARS BEFORE THE MERGER OF THE PENN-sylvania State University's Milton Hershey Medical Center and the Geisinger Health System, the medical center had established a faculty group-practice model to help it plan for a single clinical enterprise that would pool the revenue streams from both its hospital and professional practices. The merger that created the Penn State Geisinger Health System (PSGHS) took place on July 1, 1997; serendipitously, the combined hospital-physician budget was to go into effect on that same day. A full description of the merger, "The Penn State University and the Geisinger Health System: The Anatomy of a Merger," appears in the case studies in appendix A.

CHANGES IN THE OFFING

Penn State's clinical chairs were preparing for a major cultural change. Undoubtedly, the preparation considerably eased the cultural and psychological

---

Dr. Biebuyck is senior associate dean for academic affairs, College of Medicine, Pennsylvania State University.

effects of the new shared governance, compensation plans, and different budgetary practices initiated by the merger.

Among the concerns of the planners were the future roles of the College of Medicine's clinical department chairs and clinical center directors, particularly within the PSGHS. A task force assigned to explore this issue set out to answer the following questions:

1. What would be the responsibilities of the department chair?

2. What would be the joint and shared responsibilities of the clinical faculty, the department chair, the center (or service-line) director, and the group practice/health system governance?

3. Which leader in the future organization, in which responsibilities would cross traditional lines, would the clinical faculty identify with in terms of career and leadership guidance and advice?

Prior to the merger, the Penn State chairs, along with most of their colleagues nationwide, had, rightly or wrongly, developed definite perceptions of the new corporate culture creeping across academic health centers. Ronald D. Miller, MD, of the University of California, San Francisco, in a 1997 personal communication to the author, best summarized such perceptions (or fears) as stemming from changes in the following areas:

Department: Elimination of departmental structure, development of service lines, loss of financial control, and need to negotiate for positions rather than budgets.

CEO and dean: Now totally involved in directing the business of the clinical enterprise and a builder of collective decision making rather than a master of bilateral deals with the chairs.

Hospital COO: Clinical departments now seen as clinical programs offering shared risk and reward rather than allowing the accumulation of a hospital surplus.

Chair: Change from an internally directed entrepreneurial perspective to a member of institutional management, and from highly specialized academic notoriety to a macro view of success in the new clinical environment.

To those perceptions of change there were added the new, real challenges for the chair, namely:

- A need to motivate faculty to teach and conduct research while demanding ever-increasing clinical efforts.
- Changed expectations of the CEO/dean.
- The separation of academic and clinical missions and their funding streams.
- The loss of departmental autonomy.
- The loss of clinical management responsibilities.
- The increased influence in overall institutional directions through participation in group practice/clinical enterprise/health system governance.
- The addition of new prerequisites: institutional vision, adaptability, business acumen, and leadership training.
- A need for a financial definition of tenure and academic compensation.
- A need for new collegial partnerships and relationships with administrators and nurses.
- A need for subtle changes in leadership style as a majority of clinical faculty become focused solely on clinical care, i.e., as clinical effort increases, protected time decreases.

NEW ROLES FOR THE
DEPARTMENT CHAIR

Building on the differences between leadership and management tasks summarized by Kotter (1996) (table 1), the Penn State study identified fifty-seven functions of a clinical chair across the spectrum of leadership, academic management, and clinical management (table 2). The task force concluded that, in the merged clinical enterprise, all department chairs would continue to hold primary responsibilities for leadership and academic functions within their disciplines, but that clinical management responsibilities would be shared with several other leaders. In fact, some of these other leaders would hold responsibility for some of the historic duties of the chair.

What is often forgotten is that chairs truly occupy the vital interface between the executive leadership and the faculty. Not only must they accept major changes emotionally and intellectually, but they must subsequently (and in short order) lead their faculties into these new cultures—and do so with enthu-

---

Table 1
DIFFERENCES IN MANAGEMENT AND LEADERSHIP ROLES

MANAGEMENT	LEADERSHIP
Tasks	*Tasks*
Planning and budgeting	Establishing direction
Organizing and staffing	Aligning people
Controlling and problem-solving	Motivating and inspiring
Results	*Results*
Produces a degree of predictability and order and has the potential to consistently produce the short-term results expected by various stakeholders	Produces change, often to a dramatic degree, with the potential to produce extremely useful change

siasm. Indeed, theirs is perhaps the most stressful of all roles in the changing academic health center. A CEO and dean can easily change a single chair who does not become a team player in this new paradigm. (Penn State football coach Joe Paterno has said that "no organization is so fragile that it cannot afford to lose one or two non-team players!") However, the chairs themselves do not have the luxury of having a back-up bench or dealing with a small group. They must deal with large numbers of faculty and, if they are to be successful, must move their faculty into a committed and total buy-in to the new culture. And, as they exhort their faculties to understand and accept the changes in career emphasis and expectations (or entitlements), chairs are faced with a wide range of behavior (figure 1).

SETTING THE STAGE FOR CHANGE

The PSGHS merger, with its specifically identified separate clinical and academic income streams, accelerated the need for chairs to accept an academic compensation plan, the imminent demise of the era of liberal cross-subsidization of missions, and the end of the era of unfunded nonclinical time.

To motivate faculty, chairs have to understand the principles involved in leading change. Kotter (1996) has elegantly constructed an eight-stage process of creating major change, as follows:

1. Establishing a sense of urgency.
2. Creating a guiding team with enough power to lead the change.
3. Creating a vision and strategy.
4. Communicating the change vision.

5. Empowering broad-based action.

6. Generating short-term wins.

7. Consolidating gains and producing more change.

8. Institutionalizing new approaches in the culture.

It is apparent throughout the nation that the successful departmental chairs of the past few years had to have a very different intellectual focus and career trajectory than their colleagues in the 70s and 80s.

Table 2.
PRIMARY AND SHARED FUNCTIONS OF THE ACADEMIC CHAIR, PENNSYLVANIA STATE UNIVERSITY COLLEGE OF MEDICINE

LEADERSHIP	ACADEMIC MANAGEMENT	CLINICAL MANAGEMENT
Leadership	Academic administration	Clinical administration
Vision	Academic budget	Clinical budget
Mission	Education, faculty	Hospital budget
Strategic planning	Education, residents	Clinical positions
Fund-raising	Education, medical students	Business operations
Endowment	Education, continuing	Professional billing
Faculty recruitment	Interaction with other chairs	Patient care
Resident recruitment	Interaction with relevant associate deans	Faculty incentives: volume-related
Scholarship	Hospital management operations	Hospital-based physician practices
Faculty incentive: quality		Clinical pathways
Career development		Research, outcome-based
Promotion and tenure		Visibility, regional
Research, education		Visibility, local
Research, basic		Interaction with clinical chairs
Research, clinical		Interaction with COO and hospital
Visibility, national		Interaction with medical center COO
Visibility, international		Interaction with group practice and health system
Interaction with national organizations		Interaction with group practice and health system governance
Interaction with senior VP, dean, & CEO		Interaction with hospital directors
Interaction with other chairs		Interaction with nursing director
Interaction with medical center COO		Interaction with center directors
Interaction with group-practice and health system governance		Interaction with relevant associate deans
Interaction with hospital directors		
Interaction with nursing director		
Interaction with center directors		
Interaction with relevant associate deans		

Figure 1
ROGERS'S MODEL FOR INTRODUCING INNOVATION INTO AN ORGANIZATION

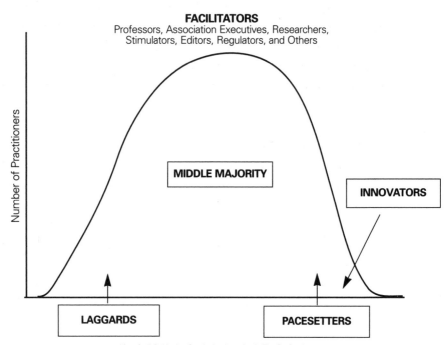

After Cyril O. Houle, *Continuing Learning In The Professions*
Source: Rogers (1983). Adapted with permission of the publishers.

Before 1992, the focus of the successful chair was on molecular medicine and answering important research questions that could lead to the development of new therapies to prevent and cure diseases. The important reading matter of the time were the *New England Journal of Medicine, Science, Nature, Lancet,* and specialty journals.

In terms of the personal career development of the chair, the emphasis was on education for an MD/PhD, basic science research, and sabbaticals.

During the period 1992 through 1998, chairs had to be concerned with the industrialization of U.S. medicine, health care financing, management of change and competition, and merger law. To keep up with changing times, reading matter today includes the *Harvard Business Review, New York Times, Wall Street Journal, New England Journal of Medicine, Journal of the American Medical Association,* and management books.

Now the career course of a chair includes an MD/MBA and a focus on clinical research and management-leadership courses. And the question that will be asked by society is whether this major diversion of many of the nation's most talented and creative minds from the advances of molecular medicine to the business of medicine served the best interests of patients, students, and disciplines during the 1990s. Certainly, some will argue that the diversion was worthwhile if it can be shown that it rescued academic medicine from being absorbed by the "industrialization" of U.S. medicine.

IMPLEMENTING CHANGE

At Penn State, such new developments as managed care, mission-based budgeting, faculty career contracts, post-tenure review, faculty accountability, performance-based compensation, and the accountability of the institution to the faculty member have all been accelerated by the merger. The PSGHS has developed different models of physician compensation, and Penn State's College of Medicine has developed and implemented an academic compensation plan rewarding academic performance of basic scientists, clinician-scientists, and clinician-educators. The plan includes a research incentive component and defines mechanisms to hold faculty accountable for the various components of academic compensation.

Salary is tied to performance in all spheres. A major component of performance analysis, obviously, is an individual faculty member's success in generating revenues and thus raising salary levels through external research grants or patient-care services. In the latter area, patient and referring-physician satisfaction, effectiveness in clinical pathway management, and patient outcomes and resource utilization are all beginning to be examined in addition to traditional approaches to physician billings, collections, and relative-value units.

Chairs justifiably question the future identification of funds for core missions. To examine their changing roles as chairs, it is essential that they assess the financial support required to fund their nonclinical missions. Data are being gathered to estimate the funding needed to address these activities (e.g., the number of full-time employed faculty required to fulfill the nonpatient-related teaching mission). This responsibility must be aligned with the other responsibilities and strategic directions of the medical school as a whole.

Chairs are appropriately concerned about identifying the sources of funds for vital, early career development of faculty—that is, until an individual acquires adequate research training to compete successfully for research funding. Thus, academic enterprise resources must be identified while the funds for the clinical enterprise are being pooled. If fewer resources are available now than in the past, it is necessary to prioritize academic missions and objectives. The PSGHS took a major step in this direction with its academic support formula.* This formula defines the limits of cross-subsidization and identifies funds for addressing non-clinical academic missions.

Penn State's adoption of the "clinic style" of career accountability in the early period of the merger will stand the university in good stead; it almost certainly is the direction in which academic medicine is going. In principle, the approach involves expecting all faculty (with the exception of those in the early career development, research-training years) to be totally accountable for each of their activities (patient care, funded research, requested education activities, and requested leadership or administrative activities). These activities, including compensation for teaching activity and performance are integral to the philosophy of mission-based budgeting, and demonstrate to faculty "the folly of rewarding A, while hoping for B" (Kern 1995)—that is, a situation in which society hopes that teachers will not neglect their teaching responsibilities but rewards them almost entirely for clinical service, research, and publications.

The merger has also accelerated Penn State's transition from some other historic faculty entitlements, a situation that many higher education institutions are struggling to handle. For example, all of our clinical faculty are now dually employed by both Pennsylvania State University and the PSGHS. This means they lose some university benefits and become eligible for other health system benefits. Traditional university one-year sabbaticals have been replaced for clinical faculty with an opportunity to apply for three- to four-month targeted study leaves. The study leaves are designed to open the way for faculty to spend time in national centers of excellence where they can gain expertise in clinical research approaches and clinical techniques aimed at supporting strategically planned directions for the health system.

---

* See "The Pennsylvania State University and the Geisinger Health System: The Anatomy of a Merger," in appendix A for details.

Certainly, the greatest challenge to chairs is maintaining the joint development of the academic health center's tripartite mission of patient care, teaching, and research in their disciplines. The British and Canadian models of small, pure academic units tied to large, pure clinical units are totally contrary to the U.S. model of the tightly linked development of both academic and clinical activities. It is this latter model that led to the spectacular successes of American academic medicine in the period 1955–1992. The danger today, however, is that our academic health centers may outsource their clinical enterprises to their own health systems, thus leaving the school of medicine with only a small group of full-time clinician-educators and NIH-funded clinician-scientists (table 3).

"It is, therefore, vital that our academic health centers retain the *team approach* to encompass joint leadership and development of *all three* missions, clinical service, research, and education. By choosing the team path instead of the working group," say Katzenbach and Smith (1993), "people commit to take the risks of conflict in order to build a common purpose, set of goals, approach, and mutual accountability. People who call themselves teams but take no such risks are at best pseudoteams. The individual components of the high-performance team are deeply committed to one another's personal growth and success" (figure 2).

CONCLUSION

Success of a merger or the creation of a large health system rests with the chairs, members of departments, and units of the health system working together

Table 3.
RESULTS OF OUTSOURCING THE CLINICAL ENTERPRISE

	Academic Health Center Academic Department	**Health System Clinical Service**
Effects on staff	Chair	Clinical director
	NIH-funded faculty	Clinicians
Effects on responsibilities	Research training	Patient care
	Research	Clinical training
	Education	Clinical administration
	Academic administration	

Figure 2
THE TEAM PERFORMANCE CURVE

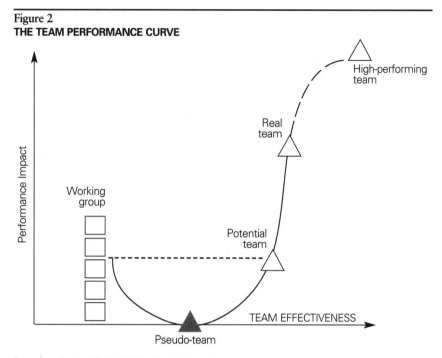

Source: Katzenbach and Smith (1993). Reprinted with permission.

as a high-performing, not pseudo, team. This performance is part of a new era for academic medicine, particularly for the academic chair.

REFERENCES

Katzenbach, J.R., and Douglas K. Smith. 1993. *The Wisdom of Teams: Creating the High Performance Organization.* Boston: Harvard Business School Press.

Kern, S. 1995. On the folly of rewarding A, While hoping for B. *Academy of Management Journal* 18:769–783.

Korn, David. 1996. Reengineering academic medical centers: Reengineering academic values? *Academic Medicine* 71:1033–1043.

Kotter, J.P. 1996. *Leading Change.* Boston: Harvard Business School Press.

Rogers, Everett M. 1983. *Diffusion of Innovations,* Fourth Edition. New York: Free Press.

Appendix A
CASE STUDIES

Cornell University Medical College

THE END OF AN ERA OF CROSS-SUBSIDIZATION OF RESEARCH

ORNELL UNIVERSITY IS A LARGE UNIVERSITY located in Ithaca, New York, with three major divisions: (1) the endowed colleges—liberal arts, sciences, and humanities; (2) the statutory colleges, which constitute one quarter of the university and include the schools of agriculture, veterinary medicine, industrial labor relations, and human ecology and are part of the State University of New York system; and (3) the medical college, located in New York City, that has only 2–3 percent of the total student population. However, Cornell's Manhattan medical campus has over 25 percent of the total research funds of the university, more than 25 percent of the total full-time faculty of the university, and, it often seems, approximately 50 percent of the problems of the university.

Cornell has a relatively small medical school with a total of 400 under-

---

This report is based on a presentation by Robert Michels, MD, then provost/medical affairs at Cornell University and dean of the Cornell University Medical College, to the Task Force on Science Policy of the Association of Academic Health Centers in Washington in 1996. Cornell University Medical College was renamed the Joan and Sanford I. Weill Medical College and Graduate School of Medical Sciences of Cornell University in 1998, shortly after this report was written.

graduate medical students, about 200 PhD students, and a very small physician program for physician assistants with 44 students.

Because the academic health center is located in New York City, it is farther from the main university campus than is typical at other university medical schools. It takes approximately four hours to get to the main campus in Ithaca by car and almost as long by airplane when total travel time to and from the airport is taken into account.

The academic health center-university relationship is important because the Ithaca campus has a very strong research tradition, including biological research in both the School of Veterinary Medicine and the School of Agriculture. Ithaca is also strong in other basic sciences. Natural alliances could be made between the two campuses in such fields as chemistry but with the campuses 200 miles apart, it is very difficult. Cornell's funding from the National Institutes of Health is divided, with one-third allotted to the Ithaca campus and two-thirds to the Manhattan medical school campus.

Medical School-Hospital Linkages

Like many Ivy League institutions, the medical school and its affiliate, The New York Hospital, are separate corporate entities. The two institutions have separate boards of directors, separate budgets, and, as recently as a few years ago, were threatening to sue each other in a local court over a variety of problems. Although the medical school and hospital share the same physical plant, the university does not own the hospital.

The New York Hospital is a large institution with a budget that is about twice the size of the medical school budget. All physicians at the hospital are Cornell faculty. The hospital is a major site of Cornell programs, and Cornell budget expenditures sometimes go to hospital-based activities. The clinical departments of the two institutions are jointly planned and funded, but their increasingly divergent missions create tensions with regard to resources.

Proximity to Other Research Centers

Another distinctive characteristic of the Cornell University Medical College is its location on a small piece of land in an exclusive area of Manhattan across the street from Rockefeller University and the Memorial Sloan-Kettering

Cancer Center, each of which has a fairly large, basic biomedical research enterprise of great distinction. Cornell has close ties with these institutions in educational programs. The three institutions jointly operate an MD-PhD program; Cornell University's medical college graduate school is operated jointly by Sloan-Kettering and Cornell. There are also several research collaborations, with varying arrangements in terms of governance, funding sources, budgeting, and indirect costs.

The three institutions have explored various ways of doing things together, particularly the development of core facilities that could be shared and operated more efficiently. The institutions now share systems for dealing with library resources, radioactive waste disposal, animal care, and tool and equipment repairs. Discussions are underway regarding sharing in the areas of industrial relations and patent activities.

RESEARCH FUNDING

The traditional academic health center has three overlapping and intertwined missions: education, research, and clinical care. The synergy of this tripartite mission has been the cornerstone of the accomplishments and greatness of these institutions. Over the last few years, there has been a strong push to separate these missions, with changes in funding and market pressures acting as the major catalysts for this shift.

As research support is constricted, science faculty want to spend less time teaching because it takes them away from what they view as their primary mission—research. With recent movement toward problem-based learning and small-group teaching, graduate students now feel that medical school teaching experience is less valuable to them than was previously the case. Those education models also make some tertiary-care oriented, full-time clinical faculty less relevant to the presumed educational missions of the medical school. However, in 1995, primary care faculty tended to be less academic and less likely to be on the full-time payroll. Clinical faculty members say they have less time for education than in the past because to earn 80 percent of what they earned last year,

---

* The following discussion employs data about the Cornell University Medical College research enterprise only. Data from the Sloan-Kettering Center are excluded because they would increase the totals by about 68 percent.

they have to spend 120 percent more time doing clinical work.

The medical school budget is about $360 million.* The faculty practice plan constitutes a little more than half of the medical school revenues and a little less than half of its expenditures. The revenues are only a little bit more than the costs. Research comprises about 25 percent of the budget, but the research revenues are a little less than the costs, so research is, in effect, cross-subsidized.

Cornell received $352.9 million in revenues in 1993–94 (figure 1), including government direct and indirect costs, private gifts, and investment income targeted for research. These revenues exceeded costs by $3.8 million. However, spending for research ($86 million) exceeded income for research by some $2 million (figure 2). (Support costs are extraordinarily high because Cornell is a research medical school in a high-cost Manhattan neighborhood.) The difference in research monies was subsidized from discretionary funds received by the medical college in that year.

The sources of the discretionary funds include monies left over after revenues were applied to the items for which they were designated or granted, investment income, unrestricted gifts, and other monies (the 5% dean's tax on the faculty practice plan). The dean's discretionary funds amounted to approximately $16.6 million out of a $350 million budget. Approximately $2.1 million went for research and $7.2 million for education. About 40 percent of discretionary funds went for such undistributed costs as those incurred by the devel-

Figure 1.
REVENUES AND COSTS, CORNELL MEDICAL SCHOOL, 1993–94

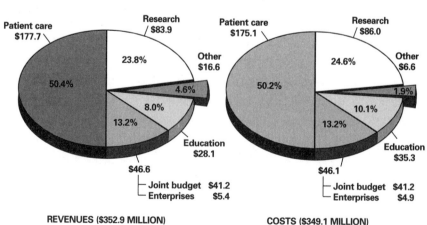

REVENUES ($352.9 MILLION)   COSTS ($349.1 MILLION)

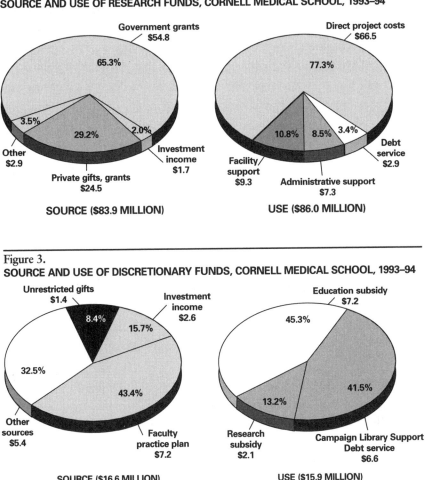

Figure 2.
SOURCE AND USE OF RESEARCH FUNDS, CORNELL MEDICAL SCHOOL, 1993–94

Government grants
$54.8
65.3%
3.5%
29.2%
2.0%
Other
$2.9
Investment income
$1.7
Private gifts, grants
$24.5

SOURCE ($83.9 MILLION)

Direct project costs
$66.5
77.3%
10.8% 8.5% 3.4%
Debt service
$2.9
Facility support
$9.3
Administrative support
$7.3

USE ($86.0 MILLION)

Figure 3.
SOURCE AND USE OF DISCRETIONARY FUNDS, CORNELL MEDICAL SCHOOL, 1993–94

Unrestricted gifts
$1.4
Investment income
$2.6
8.4%
15.7%
32.5%
43.4%
Other sources
$5.4
Faculty practice plan
$7.2

SOURCE ($16.6 MILLION)

Education subsidy
$7.2
45.3%
41.5%
13.2%
Research subsidy
$2.1
Campaign Library Support Debt service
$6.6

USE ($15.9 MILLION)

opment office, which included campaign and library support costs, and debt service (figure 3).

STAFF INCOME

The Practice Plan

The largest discretionary source for cross-subsidization are clinical faculty earnings. Total gifts to the medical school are about $45 million per year, but the dean does not have control over most of this money. About 40 percent of the base salaries of the medical school faculty come from either Federal or private research grants or contracts. However, a large proportion of faculty salaries is not included in the base. To give the institution some flexibility, some of the faculty's practice-plan income comes through supplements to their base salary. Faculty are well aware that their incomes are related to the financial situation of the practice plan. The interdepartmental pattern in the distribution of revenues has changed over the past few years with most of the loss in the very high-income specialties. To date, there has been less impact on the lower-income specialties.

About 16–17 percent of faculty practice-plan patients are currently in managed care entities, although this managed care segment is growing very rapidly. Increasingly, faculty over sixty years of age are planning early retirement, whereas five years ago they were planning to work until they died. Students and residents do not seem very troubled about the impact of these changes on their incomes; they are worried about whether or not they can get jobs. Clinical faculty between the ages of 40 and 55 are angry because the anticipated rewards are not being realized. These attitudes present a major problem for institutions. Faculty leaders in many fields are not interested in changing the structure of the system. They would rather pay lip service to how evil the change is, or write about how great the old days were, while privately discussing their retirement income.

The Cornell faculty practice plan is organized as a multispecialty, interdepartmental group. There is a 5 percent tax on the faculty practice plan to pay for institutional development. The dean gives some of these development funds back to the clinical departments for program development that emphasizes interdepartmental goals. The dean has a rough formula for distributing these funds based on the number of new patient registrations generated by each department. Therefore, funds do not go to radiology, pathology, or anesthesia, but instead are mainly distributed to medicine, pediatrics, and obstetrics-gynecology, with intermediate amounts going to the other disciplines. Departments are rewarded for what a law firm would call "rainmaking." The remaining 80 percent of the dean's tax goes to support everything else, including the basic science departments, the dean's office, the library, and the other departmental budgets.

Faculty Salaries

Each faculty member's salary is reviewed annually, taking into account his or her contribution to the institution through teaching, research, and clinical work. The assessment of productivity is made by the departmental chairperson who then recommends salaries to the dean.

Departmental Budgets

The history of the departmental budgeting strategy is one of evolution. For many years, each department at Cornell had an annual budget prescribed by the dean. Budgets were increased each year according to an across-the-board institutional formula. Every time a new chairperson was appointed to a department, a renegotiation of the base for that department took place. This renegotiation was necessary to recruit the chairperson. No serious strategic thinking about budget planning occurred except at the time of recruitment of new chairpersons. Occasionally, there were emergency appropriations, drives for special programs, or interdepartmental activities initiated by the dean. Also, gifts were sometimes given from one department to another to initiate a program. However, the basic strategy was to budget at an historic base, plus cost of living or other adjustments, with recapitalization at the time of the recruitment of new chairs. The budget appropriation came as a lump sum to the chairperson who was given considerable discretion to allocate it.

For the clinical departments, a variable, but sometimes large, portion of the departmental budget was the money received for the purchase of physician services by the hospital. The departmental chairpersons had considerable discretion over pooling general sources of available funds and spending them for departmental goals.

This budgeting system was eventually changed in an attempt to link the departmental budgets to their functions and goals—research, education, and clinical activity. The basic science departments served two of these functions: research and education, while the clinical departments served all three functions. The education budget was divided into graduate school and medical school segments. The institution developed formulas for deciding what each department would receive from the pool of research funds, based upon the indirect costs generated by each department.

In the future, the percentage of funds for indirect costs received by each department will be increased, but the department will be charged for its research space on a quasi-rental basis. This change resulted from the realization that the initial formula rewarded the squirreling away of underutilized space. In the past, even a dollar of indirect costs per square foot was worth keeping. Now, there will be a space charge for square footage, but the department will keep a larger percentage of its "excess" indirect costs.

To quantify the educational component, Cornell started with the very crude measure of classroom contact hours by the departments. Now, it is moving to a curriculum in the basic sciences that is not based within the departments, but is interdepartmental. Thus, the educational allocation can no longer be based upon departmental hours. Instead, the institution will compensate each department for its faculty's teaching time. The faculty has designed a resource-based value scale that allows appropriate recognition for various teaching activities, including preparation time and administrative work. This money does not supplement the individual faculty member's salary; instead, the administration buys the faculty member's teaching time from the department.

In summary, each department is penalized for underutilized space and rewarded for indirect cost generation, bringing new patients into the faculty practice plan, and teaching activities. Finally, to protect the stability of the academic system, Cornell decided that, if the annual allocation for any department were to decline, it could not decrease by more than 5 percent.

Initially, when Cornell switched to this formula strategy, it made a significant financial difference to only one or two departments. The formula does not save money; neither does it cost money. It is an attempt to educate the people who are spending the money about the goals for which the money is being provided. Cornell had been spending time determining the costs of its research and educational components. This effort was shifted to ensure that decision-makers experience the results of their decisions. As a result of the new strategy, it became advantageous for departments to return underutilized research space to the dean's pool and to encourage faculty to teach medical students. Both activities help increase departmental budgets. It is also advantageous to set up a primary care program in pediatrics or medicine. Even though such a program breaks even in terms of operations, it increases the appropriations to the department because it generates a lot of new patients. The new strategy is intended to provide incentives for fulfilling the school's missions.

Core vs. Departmental Research Support

Cornell devotes relatively few resources to core research support compared with departmental research support, and administrators have spent a lot of time considering the optimal ratio of such support. How many resources should be put into a research infrastructure support system—including bridge-funding for people who lose grants, basic research core support, supplements for fellows who are underfunded, and supplements to grants that are not paying full, start-up costs—and how much should go to departmental budgets?

Many of these strategies could be viewed as rearranging deck chairs; they may be important approaches but do not address fundamental issues. Cornell needs more resources and, for this purpose, has explored industrial relationships, royalties, and technology transfer offices. These types of programs usually lose money for some years before they generate results. We have not yet decided whether this is best done in collaboration with Ithaca, with our neighboring affiliates, or on our own.

We have spent some effort developing linkages between basic science and clinical departments in order to encourage cross-subsidization of basic sciences through marriages of shared interest rather than fund transfers. For example, Cornell has a program that spans pharmacology and anesthesiology and another that includes ophthalmology, cell biology, and physiology. The neuroscience program is actually embedded in the neurology and psychiatry departments rather than being a free-standing department. There are also major links between a very strong genetics program in microbiology and a very strong genetics program in medicine.

Expanding the Research Enterprise

Unlike many institutions in 1995, Cornell viewed itself as being too small in its research enterprise and needing to grow. In the last few years, Cornell has changed its planning based on such questions as: What percentage of support will an investigator in a stable state be able to generate from external sources? What is the percentage of time for which a good investigator will not be able to find funding? In effect, the institution is anticipating the need to have a higher ratio of hard resources per investigator than was assumed a few years ago. The institution also recognizes that the nature of the investigator who is considered a good investment for venture capital is changing. The economic prospects of investing in a B+/A- investigator are now viewed as extraordinarily risky. Prudent institutions are concentrating their efforts on A+ investigators.

Cornell has been actively reconsidering the optimal administrative structure of its basic science departments—even whether the institution should have basic science departments. Historically, a basic science department was an administrative unit responsible for a component of the curriculum and had a set of laboratories and investigators. But Cornell now has courses no longer structured by department but rather are interdepartmental, and the academic interests of the basic science faculty are only loosely correlated with their departmental membership.

There is much talk of mergers as another strategy for prudent expansion. There has been a long-standing interest in integrating our adjacent institutions (Cornell, Memorial Sloan-Kettering, Rockefeller). In addition, information systems make collaboration with the main campus at Ithaca more plausible than ever. Finally, there has been a very active dialogue about integrating the medical school and the hospital.

Merged clinical institutions provide an opportunity to increase the total market share for clinical services. This is the biggest potential benefit: increased resource acquisition through merger. If two medical centers in New York each have 2 percent of the market, there is a pretty good chance that, if they merge, they may be able to get 5 percent. The loser will not be one of the centers; more likely it will be the other New York clinical facilities, the health maintenance organizations and independent practice associations of hospitals, and the insurance companies competing with the two merged centers.

Mergers also affect borrowing capacity. In addition, they test the capacity to administer several systems simultaneously. Finally, leaders of the institutions must wrestle with values and institutional cultures when considering mergers. The cultural problems are tremendous unless institutions have similar missions and share common values.

Creighton University

CHANGING PARTNERS TO ENSURE THE FUTURE

CREIGHTON UNIVERSITY, FOUNDED IN 1878, WAS the first endowed Catholic college West of the Mississippi River. The university, with its academic health center, has 3,700 undergraduates and 2,900 graduate and professional students. Creighton has five professional schools and a graduate school. The university is a local not-for-profit 501(c)(3) organization with a self-perpetuating governing board. Since the mid-1960s, the board has had twenty-eight members, including Jesuits.

Creighton's academic health center consists of the schools dentistry, medicine, nursing, pharmacy, and allied health professions, plus St. Joseph Hospital, St. Joseph Center for Mental Health, Boys Town National Research Hospital, and a large multispeciality clinic. In addition, Creighton has more than twenty primary and multispeciality ambulatory care and educational sites in the community. Total enrollment in the health professions schools is 2,100, including medical residents and fellows.

The Creighton campus and St. Joseph Hospital are located in eastern Omaha, the oldest section of the city and the area with the highest concentration

---

This report is based on presentations by Richard L. O'Brien, MD, vice president for health science of Creighton University, and the Reverend Michael G. Morrison SJ, president of Creighton University, at the Forum on University Relations of the Association of Academic Health Centers held in Washington in 1995.

of poor, elderly, and minority residents. Since their founding, the university and the hospital have each been dedicated to the education, research, and service mission of academic health centers. Today, the hospital is one of the two major providers of indigent care in the community with a patient population that is about 28 percent Medicaid and 40 percent Medicare.

St. Joseph Hospital (including the Center for Mental Health) is the university's primary teaching hospital, and is currently the principal site for educating 225 residents and fellows, 454 medical students, 366 nursing students, 360 pharmacy students, 331 dental students, and 353 allied health students (occupational and physical therapists). Eight other local hospitals have affiliation agreements with Creighton for educational purposes.

Several agreements govern the relationship between Creighton and St. Joseph Hospital. An affiliation agreement sets out conditions for educating health professions students and residents as well as for other activities. The ownership of St. Joseph Hospital, St. Joseph Center for Mental Health, and a number of physician practices resides with Creighton-St. Joseph Regional Health Care System, a limited liability corporation governed by an appointed executive committee. Also governing the relationship are the agreements, signed in 1995, under which Creighton assumed partial ownership of St. Joseph Hospital and the Center for Mental Health.

The governance of the hospital rests with an executive committee with membership proportionate to ownership. St. Joseph and the Center for Mental Health each has a governing board with substantial membership designated by the university and several medical staff (faculty) members. In addition, each governing board has several members representing the Omaha community.

For almost a century, the relationships between the hospital and the university changed little. A solid foundation for cooperation had been laid as far back as 1892, when the hospital owners, the Sisters of St. Francis, agreed that the hospital would be "reserved in perpetuity for the faculty and students of the John A. Creighton Medical College."

However, beginning in the early 1970s, major social and demographic factors precipitated a change in the nature of the relationship and the eventual sale of the hospital to a for-profit, investor-owned enterprise. Coupled with these factors were the tremendous economic changes of the 1980s, particularly the prospective payment system.

This report briefly discusses the history of the university-hospital relationship, the evolution of change, and the impact of the sale of the hospital on the missions of the academic health center and the university and the implications of these developments for the future.

HISTORY OF THE HOSPITAL, 1870 TO 1983

St. Joseph Hospital in Omaha, Nebraska, was established in 1870 by the Sisters of Mercy and sold to the Sisters of St. Francis in 1880. The growth and expansion of Omaha required a new facility, which John A. Creighton built and endowed in 1892 on a new site. The new hospital, Creighton Memorial St. Joseph's Hospital, became the teaching affiliate of the John A. Creighton Medical College founded in the same year. The medical college was part of Creighton University, which had been named for John's brother and incorporated as a university in 1878.

Since its founding, the medical college has maintained its affiliation with the hospital. Currently, all staff members at St. Joseph (renamed again in 1977) hold either full-time or voluntary faculty appointments. Hospital service chiefs are school of medicine department chairpersons or division chiefs. The hospital and university are jointly involved in reviewing and selecting hospital leadership, department chairpersons, and deans.

In 1972, the advanced age of many of the Sisters of St. Francis and lack of new members in the order resulted in the transfer of ownership of the hospital to the Creighton Omaha Regional Health Care Corporation (CORHCC), a community-based charitable organization.

The 85-year-old St. Joseph facility was replaced by a new, acute care hospital that was built on the Creighton campus and opened in 1977. Contiguous with the hospital are buildings that house outpatient services, offices, and laboratories for university faculty, as well as the Boys Town National Research Hospital. The cost to construct and equip the new 431-bed hospital was $63 million, which was approximately 90 percent leveraged. The St. Joseph Center for Mental Health, a 161-bed psychiatric hospital that is an integral part of the St. Joseph and Creighton University teaching programs, is located approximately three miles from the university campus.

There are two major providers of medical residency training in Nebraska, Creighton University and the University of Nebraska; a small family-practice program at Clarkson Hospital operates independently. The universities sponsor joint residencies in psychiatry, pediatrics, orthopedics, and neurology and some fellowship programs. Residents and fellows rotate through a variety of community sites. The lack of freestanding residencies is a major factor when Creighton's administrators and faculty consider educational options and appropriate educational structures for the future.

THE CHANGING FINANCIAL PICTURE

In 1983, the new St. Joseph Hospital and the St. Joseph Center for Mental Health, which remained on the site of the old St. Joseph Hospital, had occupancy rates of approximately 90 percent and net revenues of $84 million. After all expenses, the two institutions had approximately $500,000 on the bottom line. St. Joseph Hospital had operating reserves of $7 million, expenses of $83.5 million, and debt of about $60 million. The small operating margin and operating reserves raised concern among hospital managers, the leadership of CORHCC, and the leadership of the university. The six-year-old hospital was beginning to anticipate a significant need for capital investment in maintenance, equipment replacement, and new technology development.

As a result, St. Joseph Hospital hired a consultant to guide a strategic planning process that would address the long-term needs of the institution. The planning process led to the prediction that within five to ten years the hospital would be unable to meet its capital requirements for maintenance and improvement if it continued in its current mode of operation. Administrators also recognized that the introduction of prospective payment for Medicare patients and the growth of managed care would make it difficult and complicated for the hospital to meet its capital needs.

The merger of St. Joseph Hospital with one or more other institutions was one idea that surfaced in the planning process. More specifically, merger or consolidation with a large health care system was considered as a means to achieve economies of scale, increased purchasing power, and improved access to capital. As a single hospital, access to additional borrowed capital would have been difficult given St. Joseph Hospital's substantial debt load.

In December 1983, American Medical International (AMI), an investor-owned, for-profit company, headquartered in Beverly Hills, California, made inquiries regarding the possibility of acquiring St. Joseph Hospital. This inquiry was independent of the planning process. AMI, with more than 140 hospitals throughout the United States and Europe, began discussions by giving assurances that it would continue to operate the facility as a Catholic hospital fully committed to the health professions education programs of Creighton University as well as to the Catholic health missions. It should be noted that, in 1983, Omaha did not have much activity related to building health care or hospital networks. It already had a number of community hospitals providing quality care, and some considered themselves tertiary care centers.

SALE OF THE HOSPITAL

After consideration of several alternatives, including possible alliances with some of the local hospitals, it was decided that the most feasible course of action was to negotiate the sale of St. Joseph Hospital to AMI. The parties entered into negotiations with the avowed intention of ensuring the future of St. Joseph Hospital as part of a Catholic academic health center.

The possibility of an investor-owned hospital on the Creighton University campus that would serve as the university's primary teaching hospital stirred great interest in the university community. Issues raised during the negotiations mainly related to the propriety of a for-profit, investor-owned company operating a Catholic university teaching hospital and the potential compatability of the two institutions. Ethical questions concerning for-profit health care also emerged. Among the concerns were whether AMI would support educational programs, continue to provide care for the indigent, and support a strong pastoral care program. From a religious perspective, there was concern that the AMI affiliation could be deemed as cooperation in immoral acts if certain health care practices such as abortions were permitted at other hospitals owned by the corporation.

During the negotiations, university faculty, medical staff, hospital employees, community leaders, and religious leaders were consulted and kept informed of the discussions. The proposed acquisition was widely debated. Faculty and community involvement allowed the expression of concerns and the resolution of contentious issues. After several months of negotiation, Creighton University, AMI, CORHCC, and Boys Town reached an agreement on the acquisition of St. Joseph Hospital by AMI. The openness of the process probably contributed to minimal faculty opposition.

Governance

Continued local governance was an important part of Creighton's negotiating stance and AMI appeared comfortable with this position in the negotiating process. AMI delegated a lot more authority to the local boards in Omaha than it did to other hospitals in its chain. This situation would become problematic in the future.

Under AMI ownership, the board of St. Joseph Hospital was constituted as follows: four positions elected by the medical staff; two Creighton representatives; one Boys Town representative; six community representatives; and three AMI representatives. A fourth AMI representative was added with the addition of the hospital CEO, making it a seventeen-member board. The composition and size of the board of the Center for Mental Health was similar, with two representatives from Creighton, two from Boys Town, three physician representatives (two elected and the chairman of psychiatry), six community representatives, and four people from AMI.

The St. Joseph Hospital board had remarkable authority, including the ability to hire and fire the executive director and control budgets. The board deserves significant credit for the hospital's successful operations between 1984 and 1990. AMI also played a role in this success by bringing in very efficient, top-rated administrative support systems.

Terms of the Sale

The terms of the sale included contractual commitments to operate a Catholic teaching hospital in support of the educational programs of Creighton University and to continue indigent patient care as defined by Creighton University policy. Strong local governance was established with substantial powers residing in local governing boards. A new mental health center was to be constructed, and AMI committed substantial funding for new equipment in excess of that required for replacement and maintenance.

In addition, AMI made a $3 million contribution to a new, tax-exempt foundation, the Health Future Foundation, and agreed to contribute $200,000 annually for ten years to establish a Center for the Study of Health Policy and Ethics at Creighton University. Proceeds from the sale of the hospital were deposited in the Health Future Foundation, whose beneficiaries are the Creighton health professions schools. When the sale closed, the foundation had assets of approximately $40 million.

A buy-back clause was included in the acquisition agreement under which CORHCC or Creighton University would have the right to repurchase St. Joseph Hospital with a 20 percent down payment and 80 percent financing by AMI at then-current prime interest rates, if (1) AMI changed ownership, (2) AMI breached the acquisition agreement, or (3) there was a bona fide offer to buy St. Joseph Hospital from AMI. The price in the first two instances would be the depreciated book value of the hospital; in the last instance, it would be the offer-ing price.

The sale of St. Joseph Hospital and the Center for Mental Health to AMI was completed on November 19, 1984. AMI established a division of academic health centers within its corporate structure with the strategic intent of acquiring five or six other academic health centers throughout the United States and developing feeder networks of community hospitals that would be regionally associated with them. St. Joseph Hospital was to be the flagship of a regional system. Separate governing boards were established for the acute care hospital and the Center for Mental Health. It was a positive step because the Center for Mental Health had been treated more or less as a stepchild by the board and management until that time.

AMI made significant capital investments in the first few years after the sale. A major renovation and expansion of the Center for Mental Health took place that increased the number of beds from 121 to 161. Capital was invested in technology programs, the purchase of community-based medical practices, and facility maintenance. Substantial cost reductions were achieved through the reduction of the administrative staff of the hospital, the provision of more efficient centralized services by the corporation, the divestiture of costly and inefficient support services, and the establishment of better purchasing and inventory control.

In addition to the substantial investment of funds by AMI, the Health

Future Foundation made grants of approximately $20 million from 1985 to 1990 for program expansion and new program development. During this time, the foundation also increased its corpus to approximately $65 million, permitting expansion of graduate medical education programs. By fiscal year 1990, the hospitals were generating annual revenues of nearly $30 million.

CREIGHTON UNIVERSITY-AMI RELATIONSHIPS, 1984–1990

In spite of program expansions, capital infusions, and greatly improved financial performance, all did not go well in the AMI-Creighton relationship between 1984 and 1990. The reaction of other local health care providers to AMI ownership and some of its actions was largely negative. In 1985, AMI introduced an insurance product into the Omaha market that created resentment among local insurance companies. As a consequence, Creighton faculty and AMI hospitals were excluded from participating in the expanded implementation of a preferred provider organization that they had helped a local insurance company to develop and pilot. Other hospital providers in the community asserted publicly that for-profit health care was contrary to the best interests of community and patients.

Perhaps of greater significance was the instability of AMI corporate management at the local, regional, and national levels. From 1985 to 1988, St. Joseph Hospital had six different administrators who eventually left the hospital to take other positions within or outside the corporation. Between 1985 and 1989, the hospital CEO reported to four different divisional directors. One directorship changed when the corporation revamped its strategy and closed the division of academic health centers, thus making St. Joseph Hospital part of a regional division. Finally, AMI had six different CEOs in the period 1985–1991. These frequent management changes required university and medical center personnel to devote tremendous time and effort to educate corporate leaders about academic health centers and their special missions and needs.

It became apparent that AMI was "in play" in 1988, with proposals and attempts by at least two investor groups to explore mergers, takeovers, or leveraged buy-outs. In late 1989, an announcement was made that a limited partnership had acquired AMI in a leveraged buy-out. This purchase was finally closed in early 1990. The new owners were astonished to discover the amount of local control that had been delegated to the boards of St. Joseph Hospital and the Center for Mental Health.

One of the earliest actions of the new owners was to reject the capital budget adopted by the local governing board for the 1990 fiscal year and to propose a seriously inadequate capital budget in its place. The new owners made it clear that they were not going to abide by the spirit of local control that AMI had committed to in the sale agreement and adhered to during its years of ownership. In dispute were capital expenditures, payment of direct costs of graduate medical education, the authority of the local governing boards, and the process of dispute resolution.

Because of the change of ownership and the reneging on the agreement, Creighton explored exercising its buy-back option at the depreciated book value, and engaged consultants to compute that value. This option was discussed with the new owners of AMI. Creighton's consultants concluded that the value was $93 million; an AMI consultant concluded the book value was $116 million. Unfortunately, the 1984 acquisition agreement had left room for varying interpretations of depreciation according to the accounting practice used. Discussions between the new owners and Creighton board members revealed that Creighton was a reluctant buyer and AMI a reluctant seller. An attempt was made to settle the differences between the parties. No progress was made.

In summer 1990, Creighton filed suit against AMI for breach of contract and sought to enforce the provisions of the 1984 agreement. Shortly thereafter, both parties returned to the negotiating table to see once again whether they could resolve their differences. The lawsuit was suspended and negotiations proceeded. In December 1991, Creighton University officials and the local AMI management and consultants responsible for negotiating on behalf of AMI believed they had come to an agreement that would resolve all the disputed issues. AMI wrote a check to settle graduate medical education support issues. But in the eleventh hour, yet another new management team at AMI corporate headquarters rejected the settlement. After a few aborted efforts at further negotiation, the lawsuit was reopened in spring 1992. This time, the atmosphere was charged by a counterclaim filed by AMI against Creighton University.

After two years of depositions and legal maneuverings, Creighton and

AMI entered into court-ordered mediation of their differences. During this time, it became apparent that AMI was a target for takeover by other national hospital chains. Creighton and AMI finally succeeded in negotiating settlement of their disputes in early 1995. The settlement agreement included:

- Clarification of ambiguous terms in the original acquisition agreement, particularly regarding the authority of the governing boards.
- Clear definition of the obligations of the hospitals for the financial support of graduate medical education.
- A guaranteed floor under capital investment (equal to annual depreciation).
- Dispute resolution by binding arbitration to avoid litigation.
- Purchase by Creighton University of a 26 percent interest in AMI's assets in Omaha, including the two hospitals and existing medical practices, to provide it with a stronger voice and to align the interests of Creighton and the other owners.
- Continuation of Creighton's purchase option.

The settlement agreement was signed on February 28, 1995. There were other specific operational agreements. On March 1, 1995, AMI merged with National Medical Enterprise to become the Tenet Healthcare Corporation.

Creighton University is now a 26 percent owner of a limited liability corporation. The advantages in this arrangement are threefold: (1) risk and gain sharing, (2) a strong commitment to the well-being of the hospital by the faculty, and (3) a very close functional relationship between Creighton leadership and corporate leadership. Creighton bought equity in the corporation by borrowing money from the Health Future Foundation. The loan was a subordinated debt, with earnings passed through Creighton back to the foundation. The foundation is still able to make grants by using the interest earned from Creighton's debt and other investment earnings.

During the entire process of litigation, there were no compromises with regard to the operation of St. Joseph Hospital and no adverse effects on the graduate medical education program. In fact, the number of residents increased by approximately 20 percent, largely because of the expansion of primary care positions. The hospital delivered quality patient care with obvious patient satisfaction. Like most hospitals during these years, the patient census at St. Joseph showed a decline. However, the hospital's financial performance was stable. Practice plan income, which is integral the medical school, increased by about 15 percent per year until 1992, when it flattened. This plateau was mostly attributable to the growth of managed care and changes in the market.

It should be noted that AMI never waivered in its commitment to provide indigent care and that the relationship with AMI had a positive influence on research. Grants from the Health Future Foundation permitted the expansion of Creighton's bone research and hereditary cancer research and other programs.

Faculty morale posed the greatest difficulty during these years. The lawsuit hampered good working relationships. Faculty morale was low; faculty viewed the lawsuit as an impediment to the hospital's quest for dominance in the marketplace. This situation was one of the driving forces behind acceptance of the court-ordered mediation.

LESSONS LEARNED

Some of the key lessons to be learned from this experience are as follows:

1. The institution must remain steadfast to its tripartite mission. The mission is also a key mechanism for helping educate corporate executives about academic health centers.
2. Strong local governance is important. The community not only must support and defend the academic health center or hospital mission but must also help ensure that the institution helps in meeting local needs.
3. A buy-back option is important, particularly in a rapidly changing market.
4. Access to and good relationships with the top corporate decision-makers are essential.
5. Dispute resolution mechanisms to avoid litigation are essential.

The future of the Omaha health care market is unclear. Columbia/HCA appears ready to acquire a hospital in the area. Managed care organizations are growing, further penetrating this already competitive market. Some observers expect the number of hospital beds will drop dramatically in the near future. These developments make Creighton University, St. Joseph Hospital, and the Omaha area interesting places to watch in the future.

The University of Illinois at Chicago

STRATEGIES AND STRUCTURES FOR MANAGING THE ACADEMIC HEALTH CENTER

THE UNIVERSITY OF ILLINOIS AT CHICAGO (UIC) IS the urban campus of the University of Illinois. The university's other two campuses are in Urbana-Champaign and Springfield. UIC is a level-one research university that was established in 1982 through the merger of the University of Illinois at Chicago Circle Center and the University of Illinois at the Medical Center. UIC has 15,000 undergraduates and 5,000 graduate and professional students, almost all of the latter at the academic health center. UIC graduates 1,000 health professional students annually.

The Academic Health Center

The UIC academic health center comprises the colleges of medicine, dentistry, nursing, pharmacy, associated health professions, public health, and the

This report is based on a presentation by R.K. Dieter Haussmann, PhD, vice chancellor for health services at the University of Illinois at Chicago, at the 1996 symposium, Universities and the Restructuring of Academic Health Centers, sponsored by the Association of Academic Health Centers and the Association of American Medical Colleges in San Francisco.

medical center. Most of the schools are ranked in the Top Ten in the country by their peers.

With four campuses, the College of Medicine is the largest in the country. The base campus is in Chicago with 175 students per class. Urbana, Rockford, and Peoria are branch campuses that are each twenty-five years old. All students at the branch campuses start their studies in Urbana; fifty migrate to Rockford and fifty more go to Peoria for the second, third, and fourth years of their education. Urbana retains a class of twenty-five, focused on a research track, and produces physician-scholars. Rockford is very much focused on rural medicine. It operates a family medicine residency, and has a rural medicine program that uses clinics in the outlying counties as education sites. The clinics are typically joint ventures with the county health departments. Peoria began as a very traditional medical school, but is changing to emphasize family medicine. The College of Medicine conducts $34 million in federally funded research annually, with another $15 million taking place in the other health science schools.

The UIC College of Medicine is the second largest producer of minority physicians in the country; only Howard University in Washington, DC produces more. UIC has an active outreach program, the Urban Health Program, which begins reaching inner-city students in grade school and continues through high school. The program is designed to bring students into the university and, eventually, the medical school. UIC graduates sixty to sixty-five minority physicians annually.

The University of Illinois Hospital and Clinics, a major clinical component of the academic health center located in Chicago, is the primary teaching hospital for 700 students and 900 residents. The hospital staffs 430 beds with more than 18,000 admissions, and 360,000 outpatient visits. It operates four off-site locations, including one at O'Hare airport, and a joint venture with the city of Chicago Department of Public Health at the Mile Square Health Center, a federally qualified health center in the inner city. The latter is a fairly sizable operation, with about 40,000 visits per year. The family medicine program rotates medical residents to Mile Square on a regular basis.

The university also operates a health maintenance organization (HMO) that, until recently, was organized as a plan trust. The HMO was established to provide capitated health insurance to the students on its various campuses and had an enrollment of about 14,000 in 1995. It is now a separate, university-controlled corporation, which has begun to enroll Medicaid clients.

Teaching Affiliates

UIC's major secondary teaching affiliates are the West Side Veteran's Administration (VA) Hospital, located on the western edge of the UIC campus, Michael Reese Hospital, and Christ Hospital and Medical Center. There is discussion in the VA about the VA hospital downsizing and relocating its medical and surgical inpatient services to another VA hospital affiliated with a different medical school. This would present a major problem for UIC because the VA accounts for about 20 percent of its teaching activity, particularly in UIC's department of medicine. Michael Reese Hospital is owned by Columbia/HCA. It has gone through multiple changes in leadership during the past three years, and its commitment to education is eroding rapidly. Christ Hospital is a member of the Advocate Health System, a major regional health care system. It is the most recent affiliate (1993), but has been growing in importance. There are several other hospitals involved in UIC's teaching programs, all on a much smaller scale.

Governance

Legally, the hospital is a statutory entity, that is, the university is statutorily empowered to own and operate it. The clinical medical and dental faculty are also statutorily authorized to establish and operate practice plans under the university's governance umbrella. The academic health center is subject to the usual state requirements, including the state university civil service system. Unfortunately, this can mean that the civil service system looks at a clerk who is functioning in a fairly sophisticated way in a clinic in the same way as a clerk who is functioning in the English Department of the university. Therefore, the equity of job function is often in question. There are exemptions for senior level staff, but two-thirds of medical center employees are under the civil service system. They are also unionized.

Governance is centralized. The university has a board of trustees with nine elected members. The board was to become an appointed board in January 1997. As terms expire, members will be appointed by the governor.

The academic health center works closely with the board's committee on the hospital and clinics. The vice chancellor for health services meets regularly with the chairman of the committee. These meetings have been very beneficial and productive in terms of building understanding and support for the medical center.

MANAGEMENT ISSUES

Three key elements shape the university's view and management of the academic health center: (1) the university's attempt to divest itself of the hospital in 1989; (2) the sale of Michael Reese Hospital to a for-profit enterprise; and (3) the university's commitment to the urban mission.

Financial issues were the catalysts for the university's attempt to divest itself of the hospital in 1989. For decades, the hospital's purpose was to support research and teaching. It was formally identified as the University Research and Teaching Hospital and no patient was billed until sometime in the 1970s. The university had little perspective on the management needs of a medical center enterprise, which, by the late 1980s, led to significant deficits at the hospital and inadequate revenue from physician practice to sustain the clinical faculty. Once university officials recognized the enormity of the financial problems, they responded by proposing divestiture. The university wanted to give the hospital to the county, which would manage the delivery of clinical services. The teaching and research functions would be transferred to Michael Reese, a private, not-for-profit hospital with a long, distinguished record as a community-based, free-standing teaching hospital. The plan created an uproar in the community, which ended when the state mandated that the university operate the medical center. The state then provided the institution with an additional $25 million to that end. Currently, $42 million of the university's total appropriation goes to the medical center.

Michael Reese, the hospital that played a key role in the divestiture controversy, became a for-profit institution in 1991. Since that time, it has had three different corporate owners. Currently, it is owned by Columbia/HCA. As a for-profit institution, Michael Reese has reduced support for teaching programs. Moreover, it continues to experience management and leadership problems which, from a strategic perspective, may not make it a long-term viable partner for UIC.

Finally, in recent years UIC has recommitted itself to an urban land-grant mission that focuses on public service. The concept embodied in the university's Great Cities Program orients everything the university does to the urban environment, whether the scholarly or public service activities of the faculty.

THE HEALTH CARE MARKET

In response to Chicago's changing market environment, health care providers are multiplying rapidly. Hospital systems are emerging and trying to establish integrated delivery networks that are typically oriented around medical schools. In Chicago, these systems are Northwestern Health Care Network; Advocate; Rush Health System; Columbia/HCA; two Catholic groupings; and the University of Chicago. These systems currently control 65 percent of metropolitan Chicago admissions.

Physicians are also rapidly forming groups, which are typically specialty groups or limited liability corporations. Physicians are also linking with partners to gain access to capital. These partners include Advocate, which is linked to two groups in the northern and western suburbs; the University of Chicago, which has a major primary care group; and CareMark, a physician management company that is currently very active. The physician market, which was highly diffuse some years ago, will become very well organized in the near future.

THE STRATEGIC PLAN

UIC's current strategic plan was developed in 1991 and early 1992. The institution is now in a second planning cycle, reevaluating the original plan and developing a plan for the rest of the decade. The overall goal is to enhance the institution's attractiveness to managed-care and referring physicians, which requires cost reductions in the inpatient and outpatient settings, clinical program development, and centralized contracting. A key component of UIC's strategy is to try to expand and improve its reputation. This has partially been accomplished through advertising. The medical center invested more than $3.5 million in public relations in the city of Chicago in the last two and a half years. Public opinion surveys have shown that the advertising campaigns have been successful. The community is now aware of the institution. The institution is using that survey data in its negotiations with managed care companies. For the past three years, the institution has been able to engage in single-signature contracting on any kind of business in the medical center, which has proved to be a great advantage in dealing with the managed care companies.

From a strategic perspective, the university has been focusing on five major initiatives:

1. Clinical program development—The institution decided to balance its market interest with its teaching and research missions. To this end, it is trying to focus program development to exploit and leverage existing science capabilities into leading-edge clinical services. It is hoped that community-based physicians would then value links with the activities at the medical center. It was concluded that the institution's science base made this initiative most feasible in the neurosciences, transplantation, and oncology.

2. Align the institution's clinical and academic networks—Starting in 1993, the university decided to build on educational partnerships by requiring partnerships in the clinical arena. The goal is to focus the academic resources on a limited number of partners and to exploit these academic relationships in clinical business relationships. The university has committed to a long-term strategic relationship with Advocate Health System, one of the largest networks in the Chicago area with hospitals, nursing homes, a home health agency, and two major physician groups. The significance of the relationship in the short-term is as an academic partnership, with one of the Advocate hospitals becoming a major teaching hospital. For the long-term, all of the UIC health colleges will have activities in Advocate institutions. Advocate is also the major partner for the university's Medicaid managed care product and UIC expects to participate in single-signature regionwide contracting through a physician hospital organization (PHO) that Advocate established for its institutions. That will give UIC long-term access to the market. We also expect that this strategy will provide UIC with opportunities to develop referral relationships within the Advocate system and to be the system's quaternary center for the entire market.

3. Draw clinical leadership into governance and management—UIC has

started to break down barriers between the administrative and clinical structures through the restructuring of the clinics as joint ventures between the hospital and the medical service plans. Clinicians are now in charge of the clinics with responsibilities for the bottom line. New attitudes toward operating those clinics and providing services have emerged. Clinicians have moved from treating clinics as workshops for teaching to treating them as clinical business units where attention to customer service and management of costs are vital to financial success, a prerequisite to the academic programming in the clinics. Eventually, UIC would like to expand this shared financial and operating responsibility from the clinics to the total clinical service lines.

4. Develop capital resources to improve facilities and programs—The vice chancellor for health services controls all investment dollars for the clinical enterprise, except for the dean's tax dollars. These monies are linked whenever recruitments in the College of Medicine are aligned with strategic development goals for the clinical enterprise, such as in the recruitment of a chief of hematology and oncology. A centralized system for allocating investment resources is in place, and faculty recruitment or development of new facilities and programs cannot go forward without the vice chancellor's approval.

5. Increase power and effectiveness in state relations—Single-signature contracting has been important in this regard. The state wants to move Medicaid recipients into managed care. UIC is a big Medicaid provider, with Medicaid patients representing 50 percent of its patient base. The university's HMO now has a contract with the state for 50,000 Medicaid lives at $113 per member, per month. To pursue Medicaid managed care but insulate the university from the business risks inherent in the insurance function, UIC restructured its HMO as a separate legal entity controlled by the university. The restructured HMO established a network of Medicaid providers in collaboration with Advocate. The medical center is responsible, on a full-risk capitated basis, for its Medicaid enrollees. The first enrollees entered the system in August 1996. Enrollment grew to 1,100 with almost 400 at the medical center by the end of October 1996.

Figure 1.
UIC COLLEGE OF MEDICINE REVENUE SOURCES, FY 1991 AND FY 1995

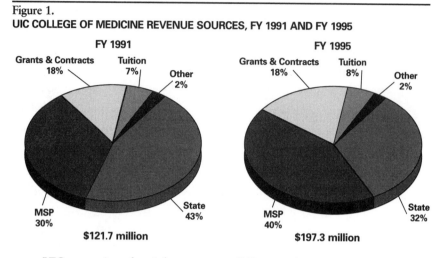

UIC recognizes that it has a responsibility to educate policy-makers and other decision-makers about health issues. It has been active in a state Academic Medical Center consortium to educate state legislators about the value of academic medicine in Illinois, including for job creation and new business development. This effort has resulted in an additional $6 million appropriation to consortium members for 1996. Finally, UIC has developed a Health Policy Center in the School of Public Health.

To facilitate the implementation of these five initiatives, UIC established the office of the vice chancellor for health services to manage the clinical business enterprise. The vice chancellor has centralized the responsibilities for financial oversight, planning, marketing, contracting, and external affairs for hospital, clinics, and the on-campus medical service plans within this office. Through this arrangement, UIC is effectively developing an integrated delivery system within, rather than outside, the university.

To ensure linkage between the academic and clinical elements of the academic health center, UIC has established a Health Services Policy Council under the chairmanship of the vice chancellor. This brings together the deans from the various health professions schools, the hospital director, the provost, and the vice chancellor for the purpose of bringing market, financial, and economic issues of the clinical enterprise to the academic side of the academic health center. The implications of developments within the clinical enterprise for the educational mission of the colleges are the focus for this group, which meets monthly. Increasingly, discussions revolve around the economics of education for the health professions within the clinical setting.

Another important organizational arrangement underpinning strategy execution is the evolution of the Medical Service Plan (MSP) from a billing mechanism into a group practice. Managed care for the MSP currently represents about 18 percent of revenue; it will be 30–35 percent in a year or two because of Medicaid. The evolution of the group practice as the driving force behind the clinical business is essential in order to attract and effectively execute managed care business. Relying on multiple departmental clinical units, even if united for contracting purposes, is highly problematic in establishing and managing the clinical protocols necessary for managed care delivery.

PROGRESS TO DATE

UIC's revenue sources experienced a dramatic shift between FY 1991 and FY 1995, with reliance on the state contributions decreasing from 43 to 32 percent and reliance on MSP earnings increasing from 30 to 40 percent (figure 1). In the same period, patient care revenues increased from $152 to $255.2 million (figure 2). Although hospital revenue has grown in terms of absolute dollars, there is a shift toward faculty practice and outpatient revenue as a percent of the total business. Managed care has had a significant impact on the clinical enterprise. Managed care, HMO, and PPO contractual relationships provide almost

Figure 2.
UIC MEDICAL CENTER PATIENT CARE REVENUE, FY 1991 AND FY 1995

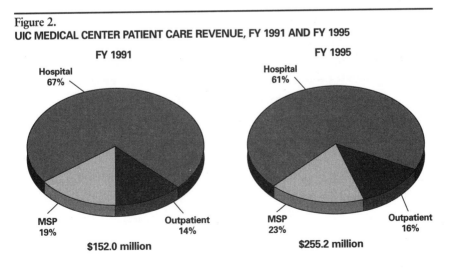

FY 1991

Hospital
67%

MSP
19%

Outpatient
14%

$152.0 million

FY 1995

Hospital
61%

MSP
23%

Outpatient
16%

$255.2 million

Figure 3.
UIC NET REVENUES BY PAYOR, FY 1991 AND FY 1995

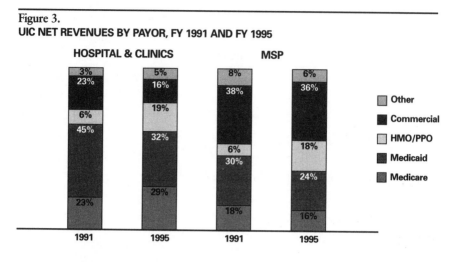

20 percent of revenue on the hospital and clinic side and 18 percent on the physician side (figure 3) and are growing rapidly. This growth has taken place even while the market in the metropolitan region has contracted.

Concerns for the Future

Four concerns are foremost as UIC looks ahead:

1. The continued evolution of the group practice into a significant business unit, and its role and participation in medical center management processes.

2. Long-term access to capital: There are no more state dollars available for capital investment on the clinical site.

3. The evolution of the strategic alliance with Advocate and the necessary adaptation of the two cultures (the medical center's academic orientation and Advocate's community-based clinical medicine orientation) to one another will bear watching.

4. Finally, the size and costs of UIC's educational programs will be on the agenda with reconfiguration a possibility for the future.

The Oregon Health Sciences University

BECOMING A PUBLIC CORPORATION

ACED WITH THREATENING CHANGES IN THE HEALTH
care environment, including increasing competition and the
growth of managed care, the Oregon Health Sciences University
(OHSU) recognized a need to achieve greater operational flexibility than Oregon law permitted in its status as a state agency. To this end, the university became a public corporation in 1995.

Prior to this date, OHSU was a state-owned and -operated public institution, governed by the Oregon State Board of Higher Education (OSBHE), the governing body for eight public colleges and universities within the Oregon State System of Higher Education (OSSHE). As part of OSSHE, OHSU administrative actions were subject to oversight and regulation by various state agencies responsible for such matters as procurement codes, property management, and personnel relations. In addition, the Oregon Legislative Assembly had to approve the entire OHSU budget, including positions not funded by state monies.

On becoming a public corporation, OHSU shed myriad government regulations that had severely hampered its ability to compete in a rapidly changing

This report was prepared in 1996 by Lois Davis, director of corporate communications of the Oregon Health Sciences University, and Peter O. Kohler, MD, president of the Oregon Health Sciences University.

managed care environment and assumed financial and operational control over its own destiny. In so doing, OHSU became the first academic health center in the nation to convert its entire academic and clinical operation from a state agency to an independent public university governed by its own board of directors.

The following discussion highlights the process of change and provides insights into the barriers to change, the major players, and the successes and problems to date that have affected the ability of the academic health center to fulfill its missions.

UNIVERSITY HISTORY AND CHARACTERISTICS

Oregon's only academic health center began as a medical school in the late 1800s. Over the years, the institution expanded to include schools of nursing and dentistry, allied health, health programs, two hospitals, a variety of research institutes, and a series of multidisciplinary units. Today, the institution employs more than 8,000 people, making it Portland's largest and Oregon's seventh largest employer. It is an economic magnet for the state, bringing in more than 150 million out-of-state dollars each year and creating tens of thousands of jobs in related industries. It has an active research program, with $200 million in current research funding. As an outgrowth of its research activities, OHSU has begun to spin off biotechnology companies, further contributing to the local and regional economies.

More than 2,600 medical, dental, nursing, and allied health students and trainees are enrolled at OHSU each year. The university's hospital and clinics offer state-of-the-art medical care. They also and serve as a primary statewide referral center for specialties ranging from primary care to Level 1 trauma services for more than 100,000 Oregonians, including a major portion of the state's indigent population.

POSITIONING THE INSTITUTION IN A CHANGING MARKET

Given its assets and capabilities, it would seem that OHSU would have been well positioned for the challenges of the rapidly changing health care environment. As a state agency, however, this was not the case. OHSU was burdened with cumbersome regulations that were not designed for an academic health center.

Efforts to position itself in the market were hampered by state contracting, purchasing, and personnel rules. Potential strategic partners were discouraged by time delays and bureaucratic procedures. State rules thwarted the university's efforts to adapt to changes in the health delivery system and to modernize its plant and equipment, both necessary to succeed in the marketplace.

Funding Issues

In addition, state support that had contributed significantly to the university's budget over the years had been steadily decreasing. In 1988, the state contributed 27 percent of OHSU's overall budget; by 1993, the percentage of total revenues contributed by the state was 13 percent and falling. Moreover, this drop in state revenues was not accompanied by a commensurate lessening of responsibility. State legislative leaders expected the university to continue providing indigent care and other public services and to finance these programs either by becoming more efficient or by increasing revenues from other sources.

Finally, OHSU, like many universities, hospitals, and health systems, was not only seeking efficiency and freedom from red tape, but also easier access to capital so it could modernize its plant and equipment. To compete in the marketplace, many health care organizations, including OHSU, need to pursue capital-intensive strategies with physicians or other institutions. Start-up funding for developing networks may be capitalized by the sponsoring hospital or health system. Depending on the size and organizational characteristics of such developments, capital requirements can be substantial.

The university could not go to the bond markets on its own; it had to go through the state and, generally, as part of a larger state bond package. The university's needs were pitted against those of other, unrelated state entities. The net effect was a $120 million and growing deferred maintenance problem and an inability to move ahead on construction projects critical to the financial future of the institution, including a modern children's hospital.

Managed Care Penetration

The Portland metropolitan area is one of the most dynamic and rapidly changing health care markets in the country. The university's service area is also among the most heavily penetrated managed care environments in the nation. And Oregon's statewide hospital inpatient use rate and hospital expenses per capita are already among the lowest in the United States. Total managed care penetration (health maintenance organizations and preferred provider organizations) exceeds two-thirds of the region's population, and HMO enrollments continue to grow. The University HealthSystem Consortium has classified Portland as a Stage IV (heavily penetrated) managed care area.

The Medicare and Medicaid populations in the state are also in managed care organizations. Nearly 50 percent of all Medicare-eligible patients participate in a managed care plan and nearly 75 percent of Medicaid-eligible patients are enrolled in the Oregon Health Plan, a state program that shifted the Medicaid population from a diagnostic related group (DRG) and discounted fee-for-service system to one of global capitation in 1994.

Market Share

In addition to OHSU's University Hospital, there are twelve general acute care hospitals in metropolitan Portland. The large concentration of hospitals limits the market share of any single facility. OHSU both competes and collaborates with the Legacy Health System, The Sisters of Providence Health System, and Kaiser Permanente, the three major health care systems in the Portland metropolitan area. As a major provider of primary through tertiary health care, OHSU competes directly for patient revenue with each of these systems. As Oregon's only academic health center, OHSU also collaborates on a wide variety of clinical, educational, and research ventures.

Past Experiences in the Marketplace

The university's experience in establishing a managed care network highlights its problems in responding to the changing marketplace. Under the Oregon Health Plan, adopted by the Oregon legislature in the early 1990s, all major hospitals and health systems treating Medicaid patients must ensure that services will be delivered under a managed care model. Many individuals receiving coverage under the new program had previously been uninsured and, therefore, had not been much sought after by community providers. When these people were insured under the plan, market strategies changed. Twenty new or revised HMOs sprang up to accommodate the newly funded patients. If OHSU, historically a major provider of services to the Medicaid population, was going to be a player in this new environment, it would have to build a managed care network from the ground up.

OHSU's ability to accomplish this task was hampered by its state agency status and further complicated because one of its key partners, a county government, had its own bureaucratic process with which to contend. However, the greatest problems came from state government. State officials informed OHSU that, to conform with state rules and regulations, the university would have to issue a separate request for proposal (RFP) for each practitioner who wanted to be included in the university's statewide network. University representatives pointed out that such a process was inconsistent with operations in the health care industry and that such a mandate would significantly delay or impede development of an OHSU network. Finally, it was noted that OHSU could effectively be closed out of the market by such a requirement.

Initially, state regulators refused to grant exemptions. The rules were waived and the issue resolved only after the university invested hundreds of hours and thousands of dollars and involved staff at all levels of the institution and the state, including the vice president and president of the university, and the governor. By then, the university was significantly behind schedule. Many providers had already been signed by OHSU's competitors, thus compromising the university's ability to build a strong, statewide provider network. In addition, the waiver the university received from state rules was only good for one year; in twelve months, it would need another exemption.

The university's effort to upgrade its outdated maternity unit also exemplified OHSU's problems. By the mid-1980s, everyone, including the Oregon legislature, agreed that OHSU needed to modernize its maternity facilities. Last upgraded in the 1950s, the unit was run-down and overcrowded. (In a facility with an annual capacity of 1,800, 2,800 babies were delivered each year.) The maternity unit also lacked basic modern facilities, with only one shower for a whole floor and inadequate space for visits by family members. Infants who required special care were transported to the neonatal intensive care unit, a full one-quarter mile away from their mothers.

Approval for construction of a new maternity facility was granted by the legislature in 1987, but the state regulatory process stood in the way. By the time university officials had worked their way through the various levels of approval and several bureaucratically inspired setbacks, eight years had elapsed. The mother-baby unit was finally opened in December 1995, long after OHSU's competitors had opened their own modern maternity facilities, thereby attracting a significant share of the maternity market. Only time will tell whether OHSU can regain a sufficient share of maternity business to support its teaching programs and contribute to the hospital's revenue stream.

STRUCTURAL CHANGES

As state revenues declined and market pressures increased, OHSU undertook a series of management initiatives to streamline operations and reduce costs. These initiatives follow:

- The administration of the University Hospital was merged with the academic administration. The position of chief financial officer of the hospital was combined with the position of vice president for finance and administration for the university, creating a single position responsible for the financial affairs of the entire institution.
- Information systems were unified into a single system.
- The hospital's billing system was fully computerized, significantly improving turnaround time on collections.
- Strategic discussions were held with community providers on ways to combine unprofitable services and to avoid unnecessary duplication.
- Medical departments were combined and/or restructured and the faculty began to organize into a single, more cohesive medical group.

OPTIONS FOR THE FUTURE

By 1991, however, it became clear that OHSU needed to take additional action. The state budgetary picture was getting worse, instead of better. The Federal picture was also threatening, with Congress attacking the funding on which OHSU and other academic health centers depended, including indirect and direct medical education reimbursements through Medicare. Managed care was growing throughout Oregon and the nation, thus threatening patient-care revenue streams.

OHSU determined that changes were needed. The first step was to assess the options. In 1991, a task force comprising representatives of the university, higher education, the legislature, the governor's office, and the private sector was convened to make recommendations about the university's future. The task force considered four options: (1) maintaining the status quo; (2) combining OHSU in some fashion with the state's public health department (the Oregon Health Division); (3) converting the university into a fully private organization; or (4) converting the university into a quasi-private organization (the public corporation model).

Maintaining the Status Quo

The first option, maintaining the status quo, was rejected as unworkable. It did not appear that OHSU could expect increases in funding from either the state or Federal governments. Without an influx of public dollars, OHSU would have to raise more revenues from clinical service, an activity that was greatly constrained by state regulation and political barriers. Although legislative leaders urged the university to do more to fund itself, individual legislators, in response to political pressures, frequently raised questions about the propriety of OHSU, a state facility, "competing" with private hospitals. (Ironically, almost all Oregon hospitals are nonprofit and nontax-paying entities.)

Combining with the Oregon Health Division

The second option, combining in some fashion with the Oregon Health Division, was similarly rejected. Although there were some areas of overlap, the missions of the two agencies were dissimilar enough that merging them would likely have led to more, not fewer problems. Furthermore, because the Health Division had more in common with traditional state agencies than with business enterprises, it was unlikely that OHSU would improve its operating agility in the marketplace by consolidating in some way with the Health Division.

Privatizing

Option three, full privatization, might have been a positive move for the hospital, but it almost surely would have created great difficulty for OHSU's academic programs and other public activities. University and state leaders were not prepared to accept such a situation. OHSU does not have a large private endowment with which to support the academic enterprise, and the hospital was not in a position to carry the full weight of the academic program.

Becoming a Public Corporation

The task force believed that option four—the public corporation—was the best choice. In Oregon, a public corporation is a unique legal entity that combines the features of a private business with a public relationship and mission. In essence, it is an independent unit of government with a specific structure, as well as rights and obligations, spelled out by the authorizing statute. Other examples of Oregon public corporations include Tri-Met Portland's transit authority, the Port of Portland, and the State Accident and Insurance Fund Corporation (the major compensation insurer for workers in the state). Each of these corporations has similarities and differences with one another. In general, they are bound by those laws that apply to all public bodies, including civil rights, antidiscrimination, and affirmative action, while not being bound by rules that apply to state agencies.

Even though public corporations are an accepted organizational structure in Oregon, not all state officials are comfortable with the concept. Some legislators and members of the state government regard these entities as too distant from conventional direct oversight and regulation by the state bureaucracy. Proponents, however, argue that the success of a public corporation is much more dependent on generation of business revenues than on tax-based revenues, thus making it appropriate and necessary that such an entity be granted independence.

THE PUBLIC CORPORATION PLAN

The task force approved the public corporation plan. However, the state was not ready to move ahead. Both the chancellor of the Oregon State System of Higher Education and the governor of Oregon decided that they were not ready to proceed. The idea was shelved for the duration of the 1993 legislative session, although a number of legislators continued to express an interest in pursuing it. Once the session was over and problems with adapting to the Oregon Health Plan and other marketplace issues began to mount, Governor Barbara Roberts reconsidered and asked that a proposal be developed to convert OHSU to a public corporation. Simultaneously, legislative leaders pushed for development of a bill that could be introduced in the 1995 legislative session. (The Oregon legislature meets every two years.)

OHSU's goal was to write the authorizing statute that would maintain the institution's public mission and character, but at the same time free it to operate in ways that more resembled practices in the business sector. To that end, the legislation clearly defined the university's obligation to provide education, patient care, research, and community outreach services and spelled out the state's obligation to assist the university financially in carrying out those missions. At the same time, the legislature exempted the university from all statutes that applied solely to state agencies, leaving in place the bulk of those that applied to all public bodies generally (e.g., affirmative action). The one notable exception was the public contracting law that applied to most public bodies, from which OHSU was specifically exempted. This exemption was critical because the contracting law had been the major barrier OHSU faced in terms of its ability to respond to the marketplace. The legislation, however, did direct the university to comply with the public policy goals of the public contracting law, including the encouragement of women- and minority-owned businesses.

Other highlights of the legislative proposal included the establishment of a seven-member board, nominated by the governor and confirmed by the state senate, to be the governing body for the institution. Instead of going through multiple levels of decision making to get programs or projects approved, OHSU could now go to this single, independent board that would be able to focus on issues unique to OHSU. By contrast, OSSHE Board had, of necessity, spent the majority of its time focused on the needs of the four-year undergraduate institutions that constituted the majority of institutions in the state higher education system.

In sum, the legislative proposal sought to move OHSU from a bureaucratically complex system to a streamlined system with a centralized decision-making structure. A link to the state was maintained by having the board appointed by the governor and by having a state appropriation help fund the educational mission. The day-to-day operations of the university, however, would have more in common with a business than with a traditional state agency.

Gaining Support

Broad support from relevant internal and external constituencies was a key element in determining the success or failure of the public corporation proposal. Within the institution, this meant working with the university's faculty senate and the two represented-employee groups, the American Federation of State, County, and Municipal Employees (AFSCME) and the Oregon Nurses Association (ONA). The faculty senate considered the plan, raising concerns about tenure, academic freedom, the continued commitment of the state to the university's public mission, and issues of self-financing for particular departments. After a lengthy, year-long process, the faculty senate approved the proposal, recognizing that OHSU needed to change to compete successfully and survive.

Although the nurses were the least enthusiastic, the represented employees also agreed to support the public corporation proposal. AFSCME leadership described the choice as being "jobs or no jobs." Public employee groups were under attack in the state legislature and they recognized that, with constrained and constricted budgets, help from the public sector was unlikely. The best bet was the public corporation, which would make OHSU better able to self-finance and maintain its job base.

The ONA was concerned that the public corporation model might not be good for the OSHU school of nursing given that it was the most heavily subsidized by public dollars of the three health professions schools—dental, nursing, and medicine. ONA would have preferred a scenario in which the state government contributed significant new funding to the institution, thus avoiding the need for business revenues. However, this was clearly not in the offing; therefore, the ONA, somewhat reluctantly, agreed to support the proposal.

Equal attention was paid to garnering external support. For more than eight years, OHSU had built a good relationship with legislators and other state decision makers by keeping them informed about the issues and problems of the institution. The university also developed a reputation for fulfilling commitments to legislators and doing the best it could with its limited resources, including streamlining and economizing when necessary. Even so, legislators needed to sign off on the actual proposal. Meetings were scheduled with legislative leaders and individual legislators around the state to gain their support. Discussions were also held with gubernatorial candidates and representatives of local governments.

Simultaneously, efforts were undertaken to build support in the business community. An advisory committee of key business leaders was convened and asked to review and make recommendations on the proposal. In the end, the special ad hoc committee unanimously endorsed the proposal and issued a report that strongly recommended approval. This report was delivered to the governor and legislative leaders.

When the Oregon legislature commenced business in January 1995, the public corporation proposal had been introduced in two separate, but nearly identical, forms by the new governor, John A. Kitzhaber, and the senate leadership. The bill was designated one of the top priorities of the senate majority caucus. It was endorsed by house leadership and widely supported by legislators from both parties. Although concerns were raised about various fine points of the bill, there was no organized opposition from any interest groups lobbying the legislature. The legislation authorizing establishment of OHSU as a public corporation (SB 2) was approved by the legislature with only three nay votes. It became law on July 1, 1995.

Despite the restructuring, several important ties between OHSU and the state remain. The OHSU board is appointed by the governor and confirmed by the state senate. The portion of the OHSU budget that comes from the state general fund appropriation must be submitted to the legislature through a budget request to the Department of Administrative Services; the same requirement holds for other public agencies.

The Oregon legislature makes an appropriation to OHSU on a biennial basis. OHSU received approximately $62 million in state appropriations in fiscal year 1995, accounting for approximately 12 percent of total current funds revenues. Of this amount, approximately $24 million was for nonsponsored patient care costs and educational support within the University Hospital and the Child Development and Rehabilitation Center and approximately $38 million was for other educational and outreach support. OHSU's appropriation from the state is budgeted at approximately $50 million per year for fiscal years 1996 and 1997.

In addition to the state appropriation, OHSU received approximately $2.8 million from lottery revenues from the state in fiscal year 1995. The state budget for fiscal years 1996 and 1997 calls for OHSU to receive approximately $1.9 million from lottery funds in each year.

As a result of its change in status to a public corporation, the OHSU board approves and directly submits OHSU's budget to the governor for inclusion in the governor's budget to the legislature after review and prioritization. OHSU also has increased access to the legislature and is able to provide direct testimony during the legislative process.

All major academic policy and program changes must be submitted to the Oregon State Board of Higher Education for approval to prevent inadvertent duplication of programs and to ensure the continuity of existing integrated programs, such as the master of public health program and the statewide nursing program. OHSU is an independent public corporation and for bond issuance purposes is treated as a political subdivision of the state. Authority for all other policy and administrative decisions are vested exclusively in the OHSU Board.

The act provides that title to the real property that was acquired prior to July 1, 1995, and constitutes OHSU's campus and certain other sites in Portland shall remain with the state and that OHSU shall have exclusive "care, custody, and control" of that property. Some question remains, however, over the interpretation of this provision and the precise nature of the university's legal interest in the property.

MANAGEMENT STRUCTURE

The president of OHSU is appointed by the OHSU board. In addition to the president, upper management consists of the director of health care systems, the vice president for finance and administration, and the provost and vice president for academic affairs, who report directly to the president.

This group is responsible for all policy decisions for OHSU. The director of health care systems, a position equivalent to a vice president, is responsible for all clinical activities, including hospitals and clinics, health plans, and health systems contracting activities. The vice president for finance and administration is responsible for all reporting and budgeting of OHSU, including all clinical, education, and research components. The vice president is also responsible for facilities management and data information systems. The provost and vice president for academic affairs is responsible for all educational and research programs of OHSU, and all the deans and institute directors report to this person. The provost and vice president for academic affairs also serves as the chief liaison with the faculty senate, which is made up of representatives of each of OHSU's educational and research units. The president relies on two major advisory groups, the Executive Committee and the University Health System Board.

The Executive Committee is made up the president, the provost and vice president for academic affairs, the vice president for finance and administration, the director of health care systems, the dean of medicine, the dean of nursing, the dean of dentistry, the director of the Vollum Institute, the director of the Child Development and Rehabilitation Center, the director of the Center for Research on Occupational and Environmental Toxicology, and the director of the Oregon Regional Primate Research Center. Major policy items, particularly those related to education and research, are discussed and approved by this group.

The University Health System (UHS) Board is chaired by the director of health care systems and is made up of the president, the vice president for finance and administration, the dean of medicine, the medical director of the university medical group (UMG), an elected representative of the executive council of the medical board, the president of the UMG, the chair of the medical board, an elected representative of the UMG executive committee, the assistant vice president of regional education, and the chief administrative officer of the university hospitals and clinics. The UHS Board plans and recommends health system strategy for final decision by the president.

EXPERIENCE TO DATE

So far, the public corporation appears to be a success. In December 1995, OHSU successfully issued a $215 million bond package backed solely by the good faith and credit of the institution. Because the bonds were sold at very favorable rates and the institution was able to tailor the package to meet its own needs, the university's annual debt payments have gone up only slightly

($500,000 a year out of the university's $500 million annual budget).

A portion of the proceeds from the Series A bonds, together with investment earnings and funds to be provided by the Oregon Health Sciences Foundation and the Doernbecher Foundation, was earmarked to make improvements to OHSU's academic, research, and clinical facilities. Some $100 million was to be applied to improve inpatient faculties, including replacing Doernbecher Children's Hospital, upgrading patient care units of University Hospital, and expanding both adult and pediatric critical care capabilities. In addition, $20 million was to be used to update laboratory areas and address deferred maintenance for OHSU's instruction and research facilities. As a state agency it would have taken years—if it could have been done at all—to obtain permission for a bond sale of this magnitude. In the meantime, OHSU would have dropped even further behind the competition.

Since July 1995, OHSU has also:

- Reached agreement—or is in the process of reaching agreement—with other area health providers on collaborative ventures that will allow all the players to streamline operations and avoid unnecessary duplication of services. One example is an agreement being finalized with Kaiser Permanente that will combine certain laboratory functions and save millions of dollars on standard laboratory tests. OHSU has also joined with hospitals and physicians statewide in Health Futures, a consortium designed to improve delivery of care through sharing of expertise and resources. While some of these arrangements were theoretically possible in OHSU's former role as a state agency, potential partners were generally much more reluctant to deal with the university then because of bureaucratic delays and inconveniences.

- Established a Human Resources Department, which brings together and consolidates personnel, benefits, employment, and other functions that had been scattered throughout campus and in a variety of state agencies. One of the first tasks of this new office was to complete a market survey of all university positions to assess the classification and compensation, including both salary and benefits, of positions relative to the community marketplace. The state personnel system, under which OHSU previously operated, did not have appropriate classifications for many health care and other OHSU positions. Therefore, many employees were lumped into an inappropriate, catchall category called management service.

- Converted the entire university to a single, biweekly payroll system, which is more efficient and cost-effective than the state's monthly payroll system. University Hospital employees had already been under this system for a few years, but the remainder of the university's employees were paid through the state system.

- Began the process of converting from a two-year to a one-year budget cycle, thus allowing the university to be more responsive to changing market and budgetary conditions. OHSU is also establishing a long-term budget and financial projection process that will project out three to five years and enhance long-range planning capabilities.

- Developed an alternative pension plan that will be less expensive than the state's pension plan, but is better designed to meet the needs of OHSU's employees. Employees can opt to stay with the old plan or shift to the new one.

- Revamped accounting processes to develop a university general ledger, which was previously handled through the state system of higher education. OHSU also is seriously considering shifting the university accounting system from a government accounting system to a more business-oriented system that could enable the university to more accurately assess financial conditions. The hospital already utilizes a business accounting system, but the academic programs have been part of OSSHE's government fund accounting system. OSSHE utilizes this system because it is required to do so as a state agency. However, the system does not work well for OHSU, a more market-sensitive institution. In a government accounting system, for example, capital is expensed versus being capitalized and depreciated as it is in the business world. The net effect is to leave decision makers with inadequate information about the cost of replacing critical equipment and facilities. A business that fails to appropriately take capital funding into account is in essence slowly going out of business.

- Commenced discussions with an insurance company about a joint project in which OHSU would hold an equity interest. As a state agency, OHSU could not hold equity interest in such a concern.

- Initiated a marketing campaign designed to inform consumers about the unique services OHSU provides. Although it is too soon to fully assess the impact of the campaign, there are a number of positive signs, including higher patient volumes and favorable reactions from the public.

While the public corporation is off to a good start, the conversion process has not been without its problems, particularly as it relates to disentangling the university from the state. A certain number of problems were predictable; others were not.

The bond issue reveals some of the bureaucratic problems that OHSU encountered. Although the legislature made clear its intent that the state would issue OHSU a long-term lease clarifying its control over the property occupied by the institution, higher education officials and representatives of the office of the Attorney General refused to issue the necessary opinions or complete the necessary documentation. Much time and money were needlessly expended before the issue was resolved. Neither the interests of the taxpayers nor the university were well served by the delay.

OHSU has also had some strained relations with its represented-employee groups. Concerns about the general job climate and a misconception that conversion to a public corporation would lead to an immediate adjustment in wages to market levels led to a brief strike by AFSCME in September 1995. Recently completed negotiations with ONA also grew tense at times. Although the strike was resolved in four days, and the ONA negotiations were settled without a strike, these experiences point out the challenge the university faces in addressing competing demands on its resources. The state deferred needed maintenance and asked its employees to forgo wage increases over the years. OHSU now faces mounting pressures to remedy these problems.

CONCLUSION

Conversion from a state agency to a public corporation may not have been an easy answer to the challenges facing OHSU, but it was deemed to be the best answer in the environment. As a public corporation, the university can respond more quickly and appropriately to changes in the health care environment, ensuring that the university stands a better chance of remaining financially viable and maintaining its public mission. The state has a statutory duty to contribute to the university's public mission. Allowing OHSU greater flexibility to operate, increased the likelihood that the institution will not become a drain on state finances, but instead will increase its economic viability and succeed in its public mission to provide important educational, research, and health care services to Oregonians.

The Pennsylvania State University and The Geisinger Health System

THE ANATOMY OF A MERGER

ARKET-DRIVEN HEALTH CARE REFORM IS A national phenomenon in the United States. Market forces have had an impact on the many components of the health care system, including physicians, physician hospital organizations, community hospitals, and health plans, as well as other organizations such as those providing long-term care and home health care. The high costs of health care have provided an incentive for employers and purchasers to reduce cost as well as choice to reduce utilization. In addition, high health care costs have provided the incentive for managed care organizations (MCOs) and insurers to reduce provider payments, utilization, and choice. Excess provider capacity in the system provides leverage for the employers and purchasers to decrease choice and leverage for the MCOs and insurers to reduce provider payment (figure 1).

The impact of market-driven health care reform and managed care upon

This report was written by C. McCollister Evarts, MD. Dr. Evarts is senior vice president for health affairs, Pennsylvania State University; dean, College of Medicine, The Pennsylvania State University; and president and chief academic officer, Penn State Geisinger Health System.

Figure 1.
MARKET-DRIVEN HEALTH CARE INCENTIVES

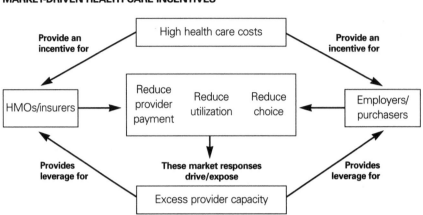

the academic health centers has been great. One of the most significant issues is on the decrease in clinical revenue that has resulted in a major decrease in the ability to subsidize the academic mission via the clinical enterprise. The long-term survival of the academic mission of research and education has been placed at great risk by such dynamics. As a consequence, academic health centers are reaching outward toward organizations such as health care systems, community hospitals, provider organizations, and other academic health centers to develop larger, broader, and more integrated health care delivery systems. During the past five years many iterations of these kinds of relationships have occurred, some successful, some not. The lessons learned to date are: The corporate world has driven health care reform; reform has accelerated the growth and impact of managed care upon all the components of the health systems; and an aggressive stock market may contribute to merger mania.

Noting the rapid growth of market-driven health care reform, and anticipating the eventual market, the leaders of Hershey Medical Center (HMC) at Penn State's College of Medicine in central Pennsylvania made a timely decision: namely, that its four core missions of patient care, education, research, and community service would best be fulfilled by developing major collaborative relationships rather than by remaining isolated in the market.

But as they evaluated potential partners, it became clear that not-for-proit organizations such as Pennsylvania Blue Shield or Capital Blue Cross had no real interest in developing a true partnership. It was equally apparent that for-profit managed care organizations such as Aetna U.S. HealthCare and HealthAmerica also had no interest and, even if they did, would not support the academic mission to any significant degree. Meanwhile, the Geisinger Health System, with seventy clinical sites throughout central and north-central Pennsylvania, was also exploring possible partnership opportunities with a number of organizations, both not for profit and for profit. For a variety of reasons, none of these opportunities matured.

A GOOD FIT

HMC and Geisinger have a similar history, culture, and missions. Each was founded as a result of the generosity and considerable involvement of donors and shared a commitment to the clinical enterprise. Geisinger, too, had a strong allegiance to education and research. At each organization, the physicians were fully employed and functioned together as a group that played a key role in making decisions and affecting change. And both had a history of strong financial performance, were interested in entering into a true partnership, and were willing to share financial risk and reward.

Relationships between the two institutions date back to the early 1970s when the two organizations created a teaching affiliation. Medical students would rotate through clerkships at the Geisinger Medical Clinic (GMC) in Danville, and Penn State College of Medicine graduates entered Geisinger residency programs. In 1987, the educational relationship was discontinued, and competition for patient services developed, particularly in Centre County where GMC is located. However, by the 1990s, the organizations again explored opportunities, none of which matured.

In August 1993, the chief executive officers and chief operating officers of the two organizations initiated a series of discussions. In December, the report *Geisinger and Hershey Medical Center Preliminary Assessment of Possible Collaboration Opportunities* by a management consulting firm was completed; in February 1995 another consultant report, *Evaluation of Potential Affiliation,* was issued. The reports analyzed possible collaborative activities and were thoroughly discussed by both organizations.

Further substantive discussions did not occur until late spring 1996, when the two CEOs decided that a team of four people from each institution should explore affiliation opportunities. The discussions began in July 1996. The teams were asked to examine the missions of each institution with an eye toward determining whether the core missions of the two organizations could be enhanced through a major collaborative relationship. In addition, the visions of both organizations, and the values and characteristics that defined their respective approaches to doing business, needed to be evaluated for commonality and potential conflict. The original teams did not use a consultant. In retrospect, this may have been very beneficial because the teams suggested recommendations that served as a basis for an organizational and governance structure that was later developed by consultants and outside legal counsel and subsequently refined by the expanded collaboration team.

The merger offered the potential of maintaining the financial viability of the College of Medicine. Among the benefits of a new, integrated delivery system anticipated by the merger was a stronger market position that could result in cost reductions and avoid imposing a greater financial burden on the parent university and the Commonwealth of Pennsylvania. The academic mission of Penn State's College of Medicine would not only be preserved but ultimately enhanced, as would the other missions of both organizations.

The geographic separation of the Danville and Hershey campuses also made consideration of a merger much easier; eighty miles apart, the two institutions did not view themselves as competitors in this era or at this time. At the same time, a merger posed certain risks. These risks included the possibility of negative reactions by providers, payors, the community, key internal stakeholders, and the governing board, as well as problems with protecting the university mission.

Establishing General Principles

At the outset of the merger process, it was apparent that certain generic principles regarding mergers needed to be followed. Thus, any resulting merger would have to

- involve the leadership of both organizations;
- derive from a common mission, vision, and values;
- be based on sound business reasoning;

- bring the two organizations together quickly;
- plan for the future; and
- monitor progress in all areas of the resulting new organization.

Because philanthropic efforts had been heavily involved in creating the two institutions and providing them with start-up funding (these are stories in and of themselves), it was critical that any merger recognize the legal obligations that both institutions had toward their respective founding trusts, the Milton S. Hershey Trust (HMC) and the Abigail A. Geisinger Trust (Geisinger Health System).

By September 1996, the original team had worked through many issues, broached the subject of merger, and proposed an innovative corporate structure. It was time to expand the team to include a broader group of leaders from each organization: the chief executive officers, the chief operating officers, representatives from the finance and legal divisions, a member from Penn State's senior staff (senior vice president for finance and business/treasurer), and several consultants.

Examining and Safeguarding Missions

Although there was great similarity between the missions of the two organizations, HMC clearly considered education and research to be equal drivers, comparable in importance to patient care and community service. Geisinger placed more emphasis on patient care and community service; however, Geisinger had maintained a large commitment to education and research since its founding in 1915. Like HMC, Geisinger believed that a balanced program of patient care, education, and research was the most effective way to improve community health. The College of Medicine's commitment to the education of health professionals, including medical and graduate students, could be seen in its sizable infrastructure. Geisinger was known for its fine residency training. Since Penn State's founding in 1967, research had played an important role in the College of Medicine. At Geisinger, the creation and ongoing support of the Weis Center for Research at Geisinger represented a significant commitment to research.

Primary care was an important focus at both organizations. At the College of Medicine, this commitment, driven by the Robert Wood Johnson Foundation's Generalist Initiative Research Grant, was evidenced in the selection of medical students with an interest in primary care, the education of primary care physicians, and a goal of graduating primary care physicians at a rate that exceeded 60 percent of the graduating class.

The opportunities for a significant collaboration were of interest to all parties. As discussions continued, excitement mounted over the vision of developing a premier, integrated academic health delivery system that would occupy a prominent position in the central region of Pennsylvania and beyond and also serve as a national model demonstrating that physician-led, not-for-profit organizations represent the future for health care.

Discussion, Negotiation, and Collaboration

One decision at the very outset was to treat the discussions in strict confidentiality. A code name was given to the project and used for all correspondence between the parties. An off-site meeting place was established for the original team, located approximately midway between Danville and Hershey (hence the code name, Pine Grove). Confidentiality was maintained throughout the process.

In late summer and early fall of 1996, the discussions took a different tack: They became less negotiating sessions and more collaborative sessions. Myriad questions emerged about a merger of this magnitude, ranging from issues of governance and structure to trust agreements and antitrust relationships. Mission, values, and vision statements also became an issue. Greg Hart, one of the consultants wrote,

> The academic mission [of Penn State] must be supported and protected in the new relationship if it is to be judged successful from Penn State's perspective. In the case of Geisinger, its core values and strategies, including those of being a physician-driven organization with a managed care strategy, must be supported and enhanced by the relationship.

The organizations moved through the process of creating what would eventually become the Pennsylvania State Geisinger Health System (PSGHS) by developing an extensive Memorandum of Agreement. One of the key features of the process was informing and educating members of the board of trustees at Penn State and the board of directors at the Geisinger Health System Foundation about developments as the discussions proceeded. At Penn State, keeping up to date on developments was accomplished through a series of individual or very small group meetings between the chief executive officer, senior vice president of health affairs and dean of the College of Medicine, the senior vice president for finance and business/treasurer, and Penn State board members. At these meetings, individual questions were answered, and a broad outline of the evolving structure and governance of the new entity was presented. The board of directors at the Geisinger Health System Foundation was kept extensively informed by its chief executive officer and board president. January 17, 1997, was set as the date for a public announcement.

Certain deal breakers emerged. From Penn State's point of view, the following conditions were deal breakers:

- Penn State must serve as the newly appointed trustee of PSGHS.
- Penn State must retain the ownership, operational authority, and financial responsibility for its College of Medicine.
- PSGHS must have an ongoing fiduciary obligation to support the College of Medicine. (Such mandatory support was critical.) The mechanism for computing the annual academic support payment included both a fixed base payment and payments reflecting a share of revenues and profit margins.
- The responsibility for PSGHS's educational and research activities must be vested in the College of Medicine. There must be a continuing role for the university in the governance of PSGHS through representation on the board of directors, and there must be an appropriate senior management role in PSGHS for the senior vice president for health affairs and dean of the College of Medicine as president and chief academic officer.
- Penn State must be granted certain reserve powers over fundamental corporate actions of the new health system (e.g., sale of significant assets, transfer of control to the parent corporation or any subsidiary) so that approval by Penn State is required for these transactions. The stipulation protects the basis of support for the College of Medicine.
- The merged entity must be in compliance with the existing trust agreement between the Milton Hershey Trust and Pennsylvania State University.

From Geisinger's vantage point, the deal breakers were as follows:

- The clinical-physician faculty of the Hershey Medical Center must be employed by both the new health system and the College of Medicine.
- The staff employed by PSGHS must be under single employment.
- PSGHS will not bear sole responsibility for the financial support of the College of Medicine; continued financial support must be received from Pennsylvania State University and other sources.
- There must be a continuing role for the Geisinger Health System in the governance of PSGHS through representation on the PSGHS board of directors.
- The initial chair of the PSGHS board of directors must be the person serving as chair of the board of directors of the Geisinger Health Foundation at the time of the merger.
- The financial support from PSGHS, as developed by the academic support formula, must be used to support the College of Medicine exclusively and was not to be available for general use within Pennsylvania State University.
- The merged entity must be in compliance with the trust agreement of the Abigail Geisinger Trust.

Other concerns surfaced for both organizations and were individually addressed. The issues included board control; executive leadership roles and responsibilities; exchange of financial details and the assumptions of liabilities; integration, including financial support between PSGHS and the College of Medicine; control of clinical operations and control of operations consistent with financial responsibilities and debt obligations of the former Geisinger organization; and location of the corporate offices.

Throughout eight months of intense and confidential planning, negotiations, and collaboration, commitment to a merger remained paramount. The leadership of both organizations participated fully in the process, consultants and legal counsel came into the discussions, and financial analyses and due diligence were begun. The activities culminated in the development of a Memorandum of Agreement and Term Sheet made public on the planned day of announcement. January 17, 1997, turned out to be the same day that the board of trustees of Pennsylvania State University and the board of directors of the Geisinger Health System Foundation voted unanimously to support the merger.

AN ORGANIZATION IS BORN

The structure created by the Memorandum of Agreement and Term Sheet* made Pennsylvania State University the successor trustee to PSGHS. The HMC Corporation was created as a subsidiary of PSGHS. The HMC clinical operations were first transferred to the corporation and then to PSGHS. Pennsylvania State University retained all hard assets. Care was taken to ensure that the obligations of the Hershey and Geisinger Trusts were met.

The key topics in the Memorandum of Agreement are as follows:

- Statement of mission and values
- Structure
- Governance
- Academic support
- Financial transaction
- Faculty and employee relations

The PSGHS Philosophy

Mission Statement—Enhancing quality of life through an integrated health service organization based on a balanced program of patient care, education, research, and community service.

Vision Statement—To be the health system of choice, advancing care through education and research.

Values—Excellence—We strive for the best, continuously improving quality in all of our activities.

Service Orientation—Our physicians and staff use their skills, creativity, energy, and loyalty as resources to provide effective, quality services in every community and each setting in which we serve.

Individual Dignity—We provide humane, compassionate, and expert care, always emphasizing the dignity of the individual.

---

*The full Memorandum of Agreement and Term Sheet are available upon request from the author at Pennsylvania State University, Milton S. Hershey Medical Center, Hershey, Pennsylvania 17033.

Teamwork—We take pride in recognizing and empowering good people who demonstrate the importance of values.

Physician Leadership—We are physician-led across our entire organization and within the many communities we serve.

Diversity—Diversity among physicians, staff, students, and volunteers promotes an environment of mutual support and respect.

Education—We believe in the intellectual and professional pursuit of new knowledge and its dissemination to colleagues, students, and the public at large as an instrument of our health system that adds value to all of our customers.

Research—We believe that basic science, clinical, community health, and health-services research advances the overall health and well-being of our patients and their communities.

Fiscal Responsibility—We exercise prudent use of all resources as part of our stewardship responsibility for fiscal and organizational success.

Tradition—We take pride in our history for it is the foundation of our future and our long-standing commitment to your health.

Driving Strategies

1. Function as an integrated, provider-led organization that is customer and community focused.
2. Service quality is the first and highest priority.
3. Managing care and improving health is the primary business strategy.
4. Advance new knowledge and innovative care by integrating research and education throughout the entire system.
5. Value employees as individuals and partners for success.
6. Population health needs and marketplace size drive clinical programs.
7. Develop collaborative relationships to better serve the health needs of the communities.

Term Sheet

A general outline of the Term Sheet is as follows:

I. Structure of Transactions
    A. Affiliation
    B. Fiduciary Obligations
    C. Names of Entities

II. Governance
    A. Board of Directors; Appointment of Chair of the Board
    B. Terms; Termination; Replacement
    C. Executive Committee
    D. Quorum: Supermajority Provisions
    E. Concurrence of Trustees Required for Certain Transfers
    F. Management
    G. Corporate Office
    H. Academic Support
    I. Faculty Practice and Income Support
    J. Dispute Resolution
    K. Advisory Board

III. Medical Staff Matters

IV. Milton S. Hershey Medical Center Trust
    A. Role of PSGHS
    B. College of Medicine
    C. Hospital and Emergency Care Facilities
    D. Name
    E. Courtesy Staff Privileges

V. Trustee Matters
    A. Term
    B. Intervention by Trustee
    C. Carryover Obligations

VI. *Employee Matters*

A. Nonfaculty Employees

B. Faculty

1. Commitment of College of Medicine Faculty Clinical Practice
2. Employment Status and Tenure; College of Medicine Faculty
3. Employment Status and Tenure; Geisinger Clinic Physicians and Scientists
4. Employment Status, Full-time Clinicians
5. Other Academic Appointments
6. Common Paymaster
7. Accountability of Faculty
8. Compensation

VII. *Management Services, Facility Lease, and Equipment and Inventory Matters*

A. Operations of Hershey Medical Center; License

B. Hershey Medical Center Facility Lease

1. Facilities to be Leased
2. Debt Service
3. Real Estate Taxes
4. Responsibility for Physical Plant
5. Utilities
6. Purchased Services
7. Program Changes

C. Equipment

D. Inventory

E. Operating Leases

VIII. *Financial Matters*

A. Transfer and Assumption of Assets and Liabilities; Compensation

B. Cost Allocation Practices

C. Audit/Review

D. Graduate Medical Education

E. Endowments

F. Academic Support

    1. Determination of Academic Support Formula

        a. Term

        b. Support of College of Medicine

        c. Computation of Formula

        d. Pre-Closing Extraordinary Events

        e. Renegotiation of Formula

        f. Deferral of Formula Payments

        g. Review of Formula

    2. Resolution of Disputes Regarding Renegotiation of Academic Support Formula

    3. Reserves

G. Research Program at Weis Research Center

    1. Transfer of Expenses

    2. Grant Income

    3. Transfer of Support

H. Intellectual Property

I. Accounts Receivable

    1. Accounts Receivable as of Closing

    2. Collection of Accounts Receivable

    3. Remittance of Accounts Receivable

    4. Costs Associated with Collection of Accounts Receivable

J. Transfer and Valuation of Hershey Medical Center Joint Venture Subsidiaries and Penn State University Community Health Center

K. Children's Hospital

L. Assumption of Assets and Liabilities

IX. *Miscellaneous*

A. New Provider Participants

B. New Health Plans/Insurers

C. Government Relations

    D. Regulatory Matters

    E. Health Benefits Option

    F. Contractual Relationships

    G. Marketing

    H. Noncompete

    I. Discontinuance of College of Medicine Operations

X. *Representations and Warranties*

Key Decision Points

Key decisions in the process include the following:

- Pennsylvania State University and the Geisinger Health System would each appoint 50 percent of the new governing board.
- The majority of employees involved in patient care would be transferred to PSGHS. The College of Medicine would continue to be maintained within Pennsylvania State University.
- Integration of the educational and research programs would occur under the leadership of the College of Medicine. The clinical physician faculty at the College of Medicine would be dually employed by the PSGHS and the College of Medicine through a "common" payment system.
- Penn State's balance sheet was to be maintained for cash, accounts receivable, physical plant, and debt.
- The HMC physical plant would be leased to PSGHS, and some HMC equipment and inventory would be sold to the new system.

Figure 2 is an overview of the resulting organizational relationships between Pennsylvania State University, trustee; the PSGHS Foundation; the executive leadership; the clinical enterprise regions; Penn State's College of Medicine; and the payors.

Critical to all the discussions was the development of an academic support formula to help support the funding of the College of Medicine. After extensive review of finances of the college, an academic support formula was developed with three components computed as follows:

    1. Fixed-base component to cover certain basic expenses of the College

Figure 2.
ORGANIZATIONAL STRUCTURE, PSGHS

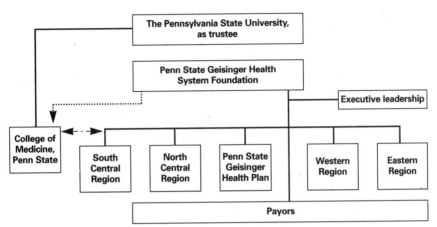

of Medicine. For the initial fiscal year, a $31,755,000 payment was made. The base amount will increase by 1.5 percent annually for years 2 through 6, and will increase at one-half the inflation rate thereafter.

2. Revenue-sharing component. An amount equal to 0.525 percent of the operating revenue of the consolidated health system entities will be included in the academic formula.

3. At-risk component. A profit-sharing component will be included that is equal to 20 percent of the amount, if any, by which the net operating margin of PSGHS exceeds the amount equal to 2.5 percent of the consolidated health system operating revenues.

Criteria were also established regarding the renegotiation of the formula and addressed the resolution of disputes surrounding any renegotiation of the academic support formula. The intent was to develop an academic formula that would meet the test of time and remain in place in perpetuity.

The scope of merged activities was significant, as demonstrated by data in table 1.

FROM COUNTDOWN TO MERGER DAY

One cannot overemphasize the number and the magnitude of the activities that occurred in the short time frame between January 17, 1997, the day the

Table 1.
SCOPE OF ACTIVITIES, HERSHEY MEDICAL CENTER & GEISINGER HEALTH SYSTEM, 1996–1997

	Geisinger	HMC	Total
Net operating revenue	$607,438,000	$380,105,000	$987,543,000
Research grants	$3,400,000	$50,697,000	$54,097,000
Licensed beds	841	504	1,345
Hospital discharges	27,309	21,418	48,727
Patient days	165,912	140,872	306,784
Clinic visits	1,450,844	416,661	1,867,505
Emergency visits	59,421	27,890	87,311
Surgical procedures	27,087	14,362	41,449
Employees	7,419	5,777	13,196
Physicians	592	376	968
Residents	202	345	547
Medical students	—	444	444

pending merger was announced, and July 1, the day the merger went into effect. Transition teams representing both organizations examined collaborative educational and research activities of the academic enterprise and discussed support systems, including information systems, materials management, human resource management, legal services, marketing, and public relations. Transition teams also started looking at clinical programs throughout the system. Little escaped their scrutiny. At the same time, the legal consultants were putting together the final documents. Along the way, faculty relations were examined, including dual employment by the College of Medicine faculty, benefits, and compensation.

Employee relations became contentious when the nurses at HMC voted to adopt the Service Employees International Union (SEIU) on April 3, 1997, and plans were made to transfer the majority of employees to PSGHS as of July 1. Again, compensation, benefits, and union issues rose to the forefront.

The senior leadership team was appointed as follows:
- Stuart Heydt, MD, chief executive officer
- C. McCollister Evarts, MD, president and chief academic officer
- Bruce H. Hamory, MD, executive vice president and chief medical officer
- Frank Trembulak, executive vice president and chief operating officer

This group began to meet weekly to reach specific agreements on systemwide functional management and to appoint systemwide senior leadership. Figure 3 illustrates the functional organization of the system that evolved.

Consultants were utilized on issues relating to management and organization; labor law; transaction; antitrust; accounting; communication; benefits; and bond counsel. The public relations units of both organizations began to act jointly, and discussions were held regarding development and fund raising for the new PSGHS as well as for Penn State's College of Medicine.

A logo (figure 4) was developed for the new health system after much discussion and consultation with marketing and public relations departments and a consultant. The logo takes advantage of the name recognition of both institutions, incorporating the Penn State shield and the red and white colors of the Geisinger Health System. This approach would subsequently permit PSGHS to build upon strong brand recognition both regionally and nationally rather than be faced with the job of marketing an unknown brand name.

Figure 3.
FUNCTIONAL OPERATING MANAGEMENT STRUCTURE, PSGHS

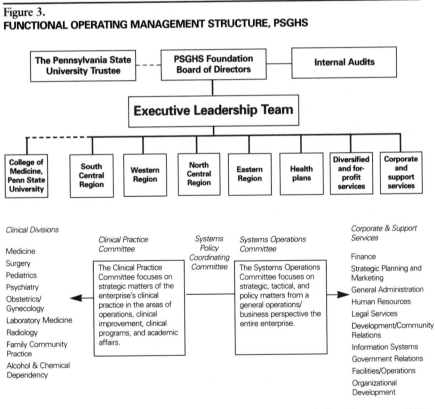

Figure 4.
THE PSGHS LOGO

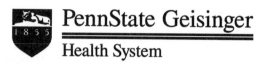

The deadline fast approached. In late June, a letter was received from the Attorney General's office of the Commonwealth of Pennsylvania. The letter requested that, in the six-month period beginning July 1, 1997, PSGHS negotiate in good faith with all health plans in a twenty-county market for contracts covering, at a minimum, all tertiary care physician or hospital services necessary for continuity of care and patient safety. The Office of the Attorney General said it would postpone a decision on whether to sue or enjoin the transaction until December 31, 1997.

POSTMERGER DEVELOPMENTS

On July 1, 1997, a new entity, the Penn State Geisinger Health System, was created. Many former employees of Penn State became employees of the new system. Negotiations between SEIU and PSGHS began, and progress was made toward achieving a contract.

The geographic scope of the system is wide (figure 5, covering forty counties divided into the North Central, Western, Eastern, and South Central Regions. The clinical enterprise is extensive, and it is the intent of PSGHS to be licensed to deliver Penn State Geisinger Health Plan's health care in all of these counties through its health maintenance organization. Indeed, in less than one year, the growth of the health plan has been remarkable—44,000 new members were added, creating the largest rural health plan in the United States for a total of 252,000 members.

In late spring 1997, the former members of the Alliance for Health, a loose alliance of three community hospitals in which HMC had been a member, decided not to consider PSGHS as a fourth partner to replace Pennsylvania State University. These relationships that Penn State had via the Alliance for Health were terminated, one illustration of the risks of a merger: negative community reaction.

Figure 5.
THE PENN STATE GEISINGER HEALTH SYSTEM, 1998

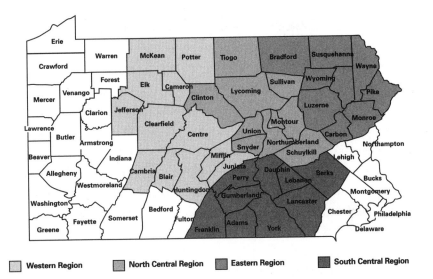

☐ **Western Region**   ▨ **North Central Region**   ▨ **Eastern Region**   ■ **South Central Region**

Since July 1, 1997, many efforts have been made to involve community hospitals in the South Central Region in discussions with the PSGHS health plan. Licensing has been obtained in Pike, Dauphin, Lancaster, and Lebanon counties, and applications made to Cumberland and Perry counties. Applications to Berks, York, Franklin, and Adams counties were also to follow.

Alexander the Great has been recognized as one of the world's greatest merger specialists. His secrets:

- Be careful when assimilating different cultures.
- Show mutual respect for values and morals.
- Adapt elements of each other's culture.
- Allow for separate cultures and identities.

And, indeed, among the challenges now facing the new system is to merge the cultures and recognize that long-term progress depends on making meaningful cultural changes throughout both organizations. This task calls for recognizing the importance of existing cultures and then layering a new culture over them that can serve as a unifying mechanism without destroying the original cultures.

Meanwhile, postmerger accomplishments and initiatives have occurred in a number of areas, as follows:

Administration

- Corporate services—payroll, human resources, accounts payable, and a uniform corporate compliance program—will service the entire system.
- Financial reconciliation and separation of clinical operations from the College of Medicine are taking place.
- Implementation of support—reporting and other functions between PSGHS and the College of Medicine—has been established.

Governance

- A single governance structure was created with the appointment of an executive leadership team, system leadership appointments, clinical division appointments, and corporate office appointments.
- The academic enterprise has integrated scientists from the Henry Hood Research Program of the Geisinger Center for Research into the College of Medicine.
- The academic enterprise increased the educational opportunities in undergraduate and graduate medical education.
- Guidelines for governance and administration of graduate medical education programs were formulated, and a Graduate Medical Education Committee and an Academic Advisory Council were formed. Also, an Academic Affairs Committee of the PSGHS Foundation Board of Directors was formed.
- Significant discussions were held regarding the annual financing of graduate medical education, workforce sizing, and annual reviews of graduate medical education programs.

Patient-Care Enterprise

- Patients gained access to a broader and more integrated delivery system with a larger network of health care providers. There has been an emphasis upon improvement in the quality of medical care as a result of case management and case protocols. Physician extenders have been better utilized.
- A strategic planning program implementation took place with an eval-

uation and revision of the PSGHS statement of its mission, vision, values, and driving strategies.

Strategic Planning

- Information technology strategy was developed.
- Teleradiology connection was made between GMC and HMC.
- Microcomputers were processed for physicians in all regions.
- A re-engineering program for human resources and materials management was implemented, and the HMC Diversity Task Force was restructured into a resource for PSGHS.
- All travel agency programs were consolidated under a systemwide relationship with Omega World Travel.
- A systemwide review program, Impressions, was developed, piloted, and implemented.
- Three CareWorks sites, which are the reconfigured system's industrial medicine programs, were opened.
- A systemwide decision support system was deployed and cost-reduction programs from both institutions were consolidated into a new program called Vision 2020.

The Penn State Geisinger Health Plan

- The South Central Region provider network grew to 855 physicians.
- Licensing took place in Pike, Lancaster, Dauphin, and Lebanon counties.
- Penn State Geisinger Health Plan payment methodologies were re-based both internally and externally.
- Negotiations with third-party payors were undertaken with HealthAmerica, Capital Blue Cross, and Highmark. A contract was signed with Health Guard, and negotiations with Aetna U.S. HealthCare were begun.
- The new Cherry Drive Penn State Geisinger Health Group building was built and occupied; a new rehabilitation hospital was opened at the Geisinger Medical Center.
- PSGHS and the College of Medicine coordinated development efforts; several major gifts were received.

CONCLUSION

In the early 1990s, the evolving market-driven health care reform environment led the leaders of two of the Commonwealth of Pennsylvania's premier health care organizations to the inevitable conclusion that remaining isolated would jeopardize fulfillment of their missions. Maintaining the status quo, they decided, would eventually result in severe decreases in revenue-streams, static patient care, fewer capital expenditures, missed opportunities for research and education, and restricted community services.

The merged health-care system they developed, the Penn State Geisinger Health System, is not for profit, in and of itself a distinguishing feature. There are no shareholders; gain-sharing is returned to the providers and the consumers. Another distinctive feature is the fact that PSGHS is provider led. Physicians occupy key leadership positions in both the new system and in the health plan. Case protocols and medical management decisions are made by the providers, not by nonproviders.

The added value of research and education is significant. PSGHS clearly recognizes the importance of education and research through the creation and maintenance of an academic support formula providing a funds flow to the Pennsylvania State University College of Medicine that will help maintain the academic integrity of the college. PSGHS recognizes that it will not survive over the longer term without a major research, education, and development component, and long-term support has been created for the "engine"—the academic health center—that drives advances in health sciences at all levels.

The Penn State Geisinger Health Plan also adds value by creating and managing the financial transactions, controlling its premium dollar, and eliminating the third-party payor. This approach will ultimately provide a marketplace advantage.

The Grand Destiny of the Penn State Geisinger Health System is to create a unique, integrated, academic health services delivery system. We have begun the journey.

ACKNOWLEDGMENTS

Many, many people participated in the merger process. These leaders from all parts of our organizations were able to look beyond the status quo to envision the future, to lead in the change and transitional processes necessary to create our new system. I am grateful to each and every one.

To the original teams, George Blankenship, MD, Mark Faulkner, Wayne Zolko, Alan Bailey, Frank Trembulak, Ted Townsend, William McBain, MD, and Charles Maxin, MD, many thanks for your innovative suggestions and setting the tone and structure for the merger. To the consultants (in particular Greg Hart and Bob Sheldon) for your open-mindedness in approaching a partnership merger unique in academic and managed care circles.

To the executive leadership team members, Drs. Stuart Heydt and Bruce Hamory and Mr. Frank Trembulak: I applaud you for your flexibility, insight, productivity, and willingness to explore new vistas.

Finally, I want to acknowledge support of the Geisinger Foundation Board of Directors and its chair, Frank Henry, and The Pennsylvania State University and its Board of Trustees and its president, Dr. Graham B. Spanier. In the final analysis they were central to the creation of the Penn State Geisinger Health System.

Rush-Presbyterian-St. Luke's Medical Center

TRANSFORMING A FREESTANDING ACADEMIC HEALTH CENTER

R USH MEDICAL COLLEGE WAS FOUNDED TWO days before the incorporation of the city of Chicago in 1837. From the beginning, it was a free-standing medical school and thus a totally academic institution. The University of Chicago came into being about fifty years later. Rush Medical College joined with the University of Chicago and became known as the Rush Medical College of the University of Chicago in the late 1800s, although no merger or other corporate relationship was arranged.

The University of Chicago, located eight miles south of Rush, became the focal point for basic science education as the importance of this element of medical education emerged in the early 1900s. By this time, the first two years of medical education were based at the University of Chicago campus and the last two years at Rush. The medical degree was granted by both institutions. By the early 1920s, the University of Chicago focused on moving the clinical years to its South Side campus. In this regard, the trustees of the University of Chicago tried to convince the Rush trustees to move Rush also, along with the Presbyterian

---

This report was based on a presentation by Leo M. Henikoff, MD, president and chief executive officer of Rush-Presbyterian-St. Luke's Medical Center, at the Association of Academic Health Centers Forum on Hospital Relations in 1997.

Hospital that had been erected in 1883 to serve the faculty of Rush Medical College.

An unwillingness to move this clinical enterprise prompted the University of Chicago to embark upon construction of clinical facilities at its South Side campus in the 1920s. By 1930, students at the University of Chicago, upon completing the two basic science years, had the option of staying at the South Side campus or completing their education at the Rush campus on the West Side. This situation was untenable in the long term, and the relationship between the University of Chicago and Rush Medical College was severed in 1942.

By 1942, the University of Illinois College of Medicine, located two blocks from the Presbyterian Hospital and the Rush Medical College on the West Side, was well established. The Rush faculty became clinical faculty at the University of Illinois and continued their educational endeavor uninterrupted, but now teaching students from the University of Illinois. As a result, Rush Medical College as a degree-granting, autonomous institution became dormant. No Rush degrees were awarded during 1942–1973.

During the late 1940s and early 1950s, the Presbyterian Hospital medical staff (the Rush faculty) continued as a major subset of the clinical faculty of the University of Illinois College of Medicine. In 1956, Presbyterian Hospital merged with St. Luke's Hospital, another major private hospital in Chicago, to form Presbyterian-St. Luke's Hospital. As a result of this merger, the St. Luke's Hospital medical staff moved to the Presbyterian-St. Luke's site upon the completion of a new Presbyterian-St. Luke's Hospital building in 1959. The new Presbyterian-St. Luke's Hospital continued its association with the University of Illinois, serving as a high-quality private hospital with a strong commitment to education. To get a staff appointment at Presbyterian-St. Luke's, one had to have a faculty appointment at the University of Illinois College of Medicine.

The major decisions that would set the direction for Rush were made in the late 1960s. Chicago, like other major U.S. cities, was in turmoil following Dr. Martin Luther King's assassination in 1968. The Near West Side, where Presbyterian-St. Luke's Hospital was located, suffered greatly from the urban unrest that ensued. Two sister medical schools elected to leave the Illinois Medical Center District (where Rush also resided) and move to suburban locations. The trustees of Rush studied the situation carefully and opted to renew their commitment to the Near West Side of Chicago, a decision that was a major factor in the dramatic renewal of this area.

In 1969, other decisions were made that laid out the blueprint for the future. When Rush Medical College had been a dormant corporation for 27 years, the trustees met annually and maintained the Rush Medical College Library, which was housed in the Presbyterian-St. Luke's Hospital. The trustees of Rush Medical College agreed to merge the dormant corporation with Presbyterian-St. Luke's Hospital to create Rush-Presbyterian-St. Luke's Medical Center in 1969.

The major objective of this new corporation was to reactivate Rush Medical College and to add other health-related colleges to create a free-standing health university. The wheels were put into motion, and Rush Medical College admitted its first students in the fall of 1971. The original class consisted of 66 students; this number was quickly increased to 90 and then 120 students per class. In 1972, the Rush College of Nursing opened, thus creating Rush University. The College of Health Sciences and the Graduate College were brought into being soon thereafter.

THE RUSH SYSTEM FOR HEALTH

In addition to the creation of a health sciences university, the vision of university leaders in the late 1960s was the creation of a vertically integrated health care delivery system with the academic health center as its focus. During that era, many experts thought that national health insurance would be instituted unless private and public institutions created a system of health care delivery that would provide care to all citizens, including the indigent. Thus, a fair share of indigent care became a guiding philosophy of the proposed Rush System for Health. It was envisioned that Rush and other academic health centers would create competing systems that would cover the entire population of Greater Chicago and obviate the need for government intervention in health care delivery. However, the other academic institutions did not see their missions as based in the health care delivery sector and did not follow suit.

Much of the credit for the vision that established the new Rush goes to Dr. James A. Campbell, its first president, and to Dr. Mark Lepper, the first dean of the reactivated Rush Medical College. Although the antecedent for the 1971 entity was the medical college, it should be noted that, since the 1920s, the institution had been primarily committed to health care delivery. Thus, the new Rush Medical College came into being not as a corporate entity unto itself but as a nonincorporated endeavor of the parent RPSLMC.

With this commitment to health care delivery, it is not surprising that the architects of the new Rush saw a great opportunity to build a vertically integrated health care delivery system with the establishment of the new Rush Medical College. It was envisioned that the affiliations with community hospitals, which in the past had addressed only resident and student medical education, could now be focused on combined clinical services as well.

With this philosophy in mind, the Rush System for Health was born with its goal of serving one and a half to two million people in the Chicago metropolitan area. It was a population-based decision, and it was assumed that three or four additional, equally sized systems would develop (and be based around other academic health centers). The assumption was that each system, including the Rush System, would care for the same number of people, or one-fourth to one-fifth of the population of the metropolitan area. Planning for the Rush System and its educational component (Rush University) was geared to the needs of that portion of the population, and the educational programs in medicine, nursing, and allied health were sized accordingly.

The decisions made in 1969 established a model that has been operating successfully for many years. The Rush System was visualized as a pyramid with primary care at its base and tertiary care at the apex (figure 1). It was assumed that all tertiary care would occur at the academic health center, with secondary levels of care at the sixteen community hospitals initially affiliated with the Rush System for Health at that time. Of significance was

---

Figure 1.
CONCEPT OF RUSH SYSTEM FOR HEALTH, 1969

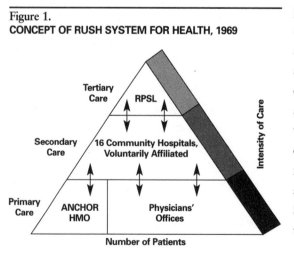

the establishment of a health maintenance organization (HMO) totally owned by the academic health center and included in the primary level of care. The HMO was established in 1970 and enrolled its first members in 1971. It is interesting to note that the original intent was to market the HMO (called ANCHOR) to the public in the Chicago metropolitan area. Although its first customers were employees of Rush and students of Rush University, from its inception the intent was to enter the insurance business in a large way. Over the following ten years, ANCHOR achieved a leading position in HMO enrollment in the Chicago area.

In the original Rush System for Health, the relationships between the community hospitals and Rush were voluntary. Each relationship was designed to accommodate both education and cooperative health care delivery activities, but not all the relationships were successful in both areas.

Corporate and Governance Structures

The corporate and governance structures, as well as the management organization of Rush and the Rush System for Health, are very simple, but the business activities are quite complex. The structures are highly centralized and closely controlled. The parent corporation is not the university, but the medical center. Rush University does not exist as a corporate structure. Instead it is a nonincorporated entity within the larger Rush-Presbyterian-St. Luke's Medical Center corporation. Similarly, the two hospitals at the downtown campus do not have a corporate structure of their own. Presbyterian-St. Luke's Hospital, with 800 beds, and the Johnston R. Bowman Health Center for the Elderly, a 176-bed geriatric acute and subacute care hospital, are operated by the Rush-Presbyterian-St. Luke's Medical Center corporation. Since its inception, the parent corporation has had a physician as its president and CEO. The same person is also president and chairman of the board of the Rush System for Health Corporation established in 1995.

Within the Rush-Presbyterian-St.Luke's Medical Center corporation are two senior vice presidents. The senior vice president for corporate and hospital affairs has the responsibility for management of the two downtown hospitals in addition to other corporate functions. This person is in fact (but not name) the head of Presbyterian-St. Luke's Hospital. The senior vice president for corporate and external affairs is liaison to the Rush System for Health. A number of the support departments of the parent corporation report to this position.

Until 1993, Rush Health Plans was a subsidiary corporation as well. Rush Health Plans at that time included ANCHOR (a staff-model HMO), a preferred physicians organization, and an independent physicians association. However, in 1993 Rush merged its health plans with those of the Prudential Insurance Company of America to form a new joint venture called the Rush Prudential Health Plans, which is a fifty-fifty partnership. Rush Health Plans and Prudential's HMO and health insurance business in the Chicago area were merged in their entireties in this joint venture, which is not a subsidiary of either organization.

Throughout the organization the practitioner-teacher model, so often used in medicine, has been employed in many disciplines. For example, the chairperson of the department of nutrition within the College of Health Sciences has management responsibility for all food services in the medical center, including service for patients, faculty, employees, and visitors. Similarly, the senior vice president for corporate and hospital affairs has held the position of chairperson of the department of health systems management within the College of Health Sciences. The chairpersons of the departments of speech pathology and audiology have management responsibilities for these clinical functions in the medical center. The same is true for occupational therapy and medical physics. In each of these circumstances departmental faculty carry both clinical and educational responsibilities.

A Turning Point: The 1984 Strategic Plan

With a change in the presidency of the medical center in 1984, a review and planning process was initiated with both a special trustee committee and senior management participating. The first question was whether a vertically integrated health care delivery system, the original concept focused on an academic health center, was still valid. The answer was a resounding "yes"! The second question was whether the structure for implementation of that concept was successful in its thirteen-year history and whether there was need for alteration.

Two problems with the implementation strategy were recognized at that time. First, there was evidence of "scatter" in the system, that is, patients were not being contained within the system but were being referred to other institutions for various services. The vertical nature of this system with patient referral both up and down the ladder of services was working well in some disciplines, but it was virtually nonexistent in others. It was apparent that stronger glue was necessary to hold the system together so that there

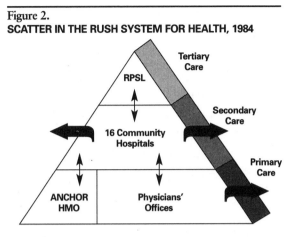

Figure 2.
SCATTER IN THE RUSH SYSTEM FOR HEALTH, 1984

would be greater incentives to function as a true system. In addition, the environment had changed since 1969, with tertiary care now provided in sophisticated community hospitals that had grown in capabilities over the period and were important competitors in the marketplace. A geographic imperative for decentralization of some of the tertiary services in the Rush System had emerged (figure 2).

A single solution, the corporate integration of partners in the Rush System for Health, seemed to solve these problems in a positive way. With corporate integration and the combining of financials, there was more incentive for the various partners in the system to use system resources. In addition, combining bottom lines and the irrevocable nature of these relationships resulted in an incentive for the academic health center to decentralize some of its tertiary services to its corporately integrated partners to respond to the geographic demands of the marketplace.

Centers of Excellence

As a second outcome of the 1984–85 strategic planning, it was decided to create a series of centers of excellence that have come to be known as the Rush Institutes. The strategic planning process, although highlighting the quality of care delivered by the various institutions in Chicago, also noted the lack of nationally recognized centers of excellence in patient care. Thus, Rush decided that these institutes would be strongly committed to research as well as health care delivery. On the health care side, the institutes were designed as ambulatory tertiary centers or one-stop shopping institutes. They brought together all of the disciplines to focus on a particular series of disease entities, usually organized by organ system. On the research side, the approach was multidisciplinary as well. The seven institutes are the Rush Institute on Aging, the Rush Institute for Arthritis and Orthopedics, the Rush Cancer Institute, the Rush Heart Institute, the Rush Institute for Mental Well-Being, the Rush Neuroscience Institute, and the Rush Primary Care Institute.

The creation of seven institutes with an equally strong focus on research and health care delivery was a large task to undertake and perhaps was unprecedented. A concomitant decision was made to conduct a capital campaign, targeted at $160 million, with $68 million designated for people and programs (not facilities) in the various institutes. A target to increase the number of endowed chairs to seventy-five was also set. By the time the campaign drew to a close at the end of 1996, it had exceeded $220 million in philanthropy and closed out the year with eighty endowed chairs in Rush University.

As tertiary ambulatory care centers, the care delivery components of the institutes were designed to be replicated throughout the Rush System for Health at the corporately integrated partner institutions. This goal is being achieved selectively in terms of both institutes and specific affiliated partner institutions. An individual can receive services from the Rush Cancer Institute from Riverside Hospital and Medical Center sixty-five miles to the south in Kankakee, forty-five miles to the west in Aurora at Rush Copley Medical Center, or twenty-five miles to the northwest at Holy Family Medical Center in Des Plaines.

When a new structure is brought into being in an academic environment, there is much consternation. The institute structure has different meanings in different academic health centers. It was not the intent at Rush to replace or weaken the departmental structure by the creation of these institutes. Rather they were seen as vehicles to enhance multidisciplinary approaches to patient care and to research. The creation of the institutes also enabled the broadening of stewardship for the institution from the lay leadership in the Chicago community. Leadership committees were created for each of the institutes; they were chaired by members of the Board of Trustees, but included membership from outside of the Rush board. These committees proved to be wonderful vehicles to broaden support for the institution in the community as well as for fund raising for the campaign.

Given the institutional respect for maintaining the integrity and authority of the departmental structure, the institutes were not given faculty appointment or tenure-granting powers. The institutes do control resources in terms of salaries and clinical and research space, thus possessing the needed authority to conduct their missions. Since the institutes are multidisciplinary and the disciplines cut across colleges (nursing, allied health, medicine), the institute directors report to the president and CEO. However, the operating relationship is so dominated by the College of Medicine that the president has included the dean of the College of Medicine in that reporting structure. Institute directors in some instances chair corresponding departments in the College of Medicine. In some instances they do not.

The maturation of Rush University was the third major strategy that emanated from the strategic planning process of 1984-85. Rush University was only twelve years old at that time. Although a powerhouse in the Chicago health care delivery scene, in truth, Rush was still a fledgling university in the research domain. Particular attention was focused on achievement in the research arena, and, over the last fourteen years, that success has been forthcoming. In 1996, Rush received $41 million in externally awarded research grants, giving it respected standing among health science centers around the country. Its growth rate continues to be between 15 and 20 percent per year in total external research funds, with growth in funded research from the National Institutes of Health at that level or higher.

THE RUSH SYSTEM FOR HEALTH CORPORATION

From its inception until 1987, the Rush System for Health consisted of a voluntary relationship between a number of community hospitals and the academic health center. Then, in 1987, the first two corporately integrated affiliates were added; subsequently six more hospitals were added in this manner, with system hospitals now totaling ten (including Rush's two downtown facilities). Each was a bilateral relationship, with the academic health center a corporate structure based upon a "bridge board" controlled by RPSLMC and the sole cor-

Figure 3.
RUSH SYSTEM FOR HEALTH, 1987

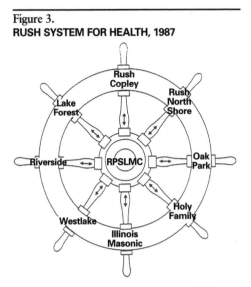

porate member of the affiliate hospital board.

The affiliate hospital board remained in place, with two more members from the Rush board added. For reciprocity, two members of the affiliate hospital board were appointed to the board of RPSLMC. The two Catholic hospitals added to the system were the exception to this structure. In these instances, the medical center became a joint venture partner in the two hospitals. Thus, the Rush System for Health was a series of bilateral arrangements that could be represented as a wheel, with RPSLMC serving as the hub and the affiliates extending from the hub as spokes (figure 3).

To address the managed care environment, another corporation was needed. The Rush System for Health Corporation was established in 1995. The bilateral, corporately integrated arrangements with each of the hospitals addressed program and facility development and education. The Rush System for Health Corporation, on the other hand, addressed those needs that could only be handled by a multimember corporation, including joint purchasing, joint marketing, managed care contracting as a system through a super-physician hospital organization, systemwide quality assurance, and the development of systemwide clinical programs. A systemwide information system is also under development.

In concept, the Rush System for Health Corporation has gone from serving as the hub of a wheel to becoming the wheel itself, thereby connecting all of the spokes to each other (figure 4). By agreement, the president and CEO of Rush-Presbyterian-St. Luke's Medical Center is the chairman and president of the Rush System for Health Corporation. However, the Rush System for Health is a one-member, one-vote entity in which Rush-Presbyterian-St. Luke's Medical Center participates on an equal basis with the other member institutions. In addition to his role in the Rush System for Health Corporation, the president and

Figure 4.
RUSH SYSTEM FOR HEALTH CORPORATION, 1987

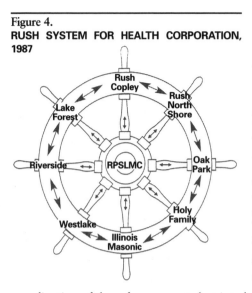

CEO of Rush-Presbyterian-St. Luke's Medical Center is also president of Rush University and alternates chairmanship of the board of Rush Prudential Health Plans with his counterpart from the Prudential Insurance Company of America. Thus, responsibility for the medical center, the academic programs, the Rush System for Health, and the insurance company is centralized in one individual. This centralization has been important in the coordination of these four separate but interlocking activities.

Staff of the Rush System for Health include the chief operating officer/ executive director, an assistant director, a director of purchasing, a director of marketing, and a vice president for physician network development. The Board of Directors for the Rush System for Health is composed of the CEOs of each of the member institutions. In addition, there is a System Advisory Board under the chairmanship of the chairman of the Board of Trustees of Rush-Presbyterian-St. Luke's Medical Center. The System Advisory Board has three members from each institution, including the chairman of the board, the CEO, and a physician selected by the CEO. The System Advisory Board is in fact the functioning governing board because of the nature of its composition. Reporting to the System Advisory Board are three councils, as follows:

1. The Operations Council comprising the chief operating officer of each member institution. Its function is to implement the business programs as determined by the System Advisory Board and the System Board.

2. The Clinical Council comprising two physicians from each member institution. This council has authority over all clinical matters addressed by the system, such as systemwide clinical guidelines, the commitment of physicians to a systemwide formulary, quality assurance and clinical programs.

3. The Academic Council comprising the deans, assistant deans, and associate deans at Rush University and hospitals throughout the system. An associate dean is appointed in each system hospital where academic programs of Rush University are conducted. Most often that individual is the vice president for medical affairs of the affiliate. Thus, the Academic Council, in contrast to the Operations Council and the Clinical Council, is heavily weighted with individuals from the academic health center, and rightly so because of the focus of the academic programs at the academic health center. The dean of Rush Medical College chairs the Academic Council and is also an ex officio member of the System Advisory Board.

The Rush System for Health has a large number of committees that report to one of the three councils. These committees are composed of individuals with comparable functional responsibilities from institutions across the system. Included are committees for information systems, pharmacy, the laboratory, and home health.

Since its incorporation in 1995, the Rush System for Health has consolidated its individual hospice programs into a new independent corporation, The Rush Hospice Partners, which provides services throughout Greater Chicago. This corporation reports to the Rush System for Health. A similar consolidation of home care services is in progress. Currently, it is not advantageous to remove these activities from the individual hospitals because of the current Medicare reimbursement structure. However, it is anticipated that Medicare rules will be changed, at which point the Rush System for Health is prepared to consolidate home health into a similar single independent corporation.

The Rush System for Health now includes the three core components of

Figure 5.
RUSH SYSTEM FOR HEALTH, 1996

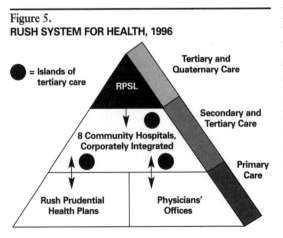

● = Islands of tertiary care

RPSL

Tertiary and Quaternary Care

Secondary and Tertiary Care

8 Community Hospitals, Corporately Integrated

Primary Care

Rush Prudential Health Plans

Physicians' Offices

Rush-Presbyterian-St. Luke's Medical Center. These are Presbyterian-St. Luke's Hospital, Johnston R. Bowman Health Center for the Elderly, and Rush University. Also included are eight other hospitals with a service area 120 miles long and 60 miles wide (figures 5 and 6). In addition, it has consolidated its hospice programs into a single corporation, the Rush Hospice Partners. Its home health programs are also being consolidated into a single entity. Rush Occupational Health Centers cover the same geographic area as does a Rush program in behavioral health (substance abuse). The system has $1.8 billion in revenues, 3,500 beds, 700 long-term care beds, and employs approximately 20,000 peo-

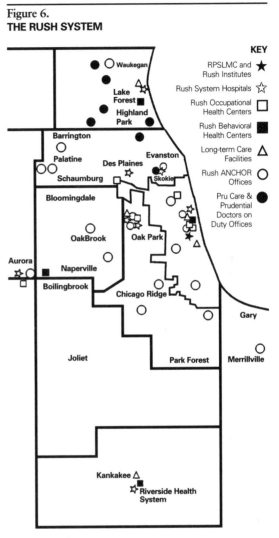

Figure 6.
THE RUSH SYSTEM

KEY

RPSLMC and Rush Institutes ★
Rush System Hospitals ☆
Rush Occupational Health Centers ☐
Rush Behavioral Health Centers ■
Long-term Care Facilities △
Rush ANCHOR Offices ○
Pru Care & Prudential Doctors on Duty Offices ●

ple, making it one of the largest employers in Chicago. The Rush Prudential Health Plans cover 350,000 people in the Chicago metropolitan area.

Rush University remains the entity with primary responsibility for the education mission. Included in this operation are more than 600 residency and fellowship positions that cover essentially all of the disciplines in medicine and surgery. A strong national program of continuing medical education emanates from the institution as well. The research component continues to be a targeted area for investment by the medical center, with a new research area of ten floors scheduled for construction within the year.

Added to the traditional education, research, and service missions, the medical center's fourth mission is community service. There has traditionally been a strong commitment to community service by the institution and, indeed, that commitment was responsible for its early decision to remain on the West Side of Chicago when other health care providers left in the 1960s. The community services are extensive and include education and health care delivery as well as research on delivery of services to an inner-city community. Of particular note is that community service has been incorporated into the curriculums of all health professions schools at Rush University. The impact of community service and its influence on career choice is currently being studied. Preliminary data indicate that students most active in community service have a significantly higher incidence of selecting primary care disciplines for the professional careers.

The Rush System for Health was designed to be geographically comprehensive across the greater Chicago metropolitan area. Through the ten member hospitals and their outreach facilities, the goal is to ensure that the population of eight million has ready access to Rush System care, with primary care capability no more than fifteen minutes from any resident of the area. The system is nearly complete; it is anticipated that three or four additional facilities will be needed to provide the desired coverage.

Rush Prudential Health Plans and ArcVentures

Rush Prudential Health Plans has a board of ten, five appointed by Rush and five by Prudential. However, there are only two voting members: the president/CEO of Rush and the designee of the Prudential Insurance Company of America. The chair alternates between Rush and Prudential.

Even though Rush is a 50-percent partner in one of Chicago's largest managed care companies, the system strategy is not to be dependent upon Rush Prudential for its covered lives, but rather to be a provider of choice for all insurers in the Chicago marketplace. To date, Rush's arrangement with Rush Prudential has not impaired its relations with other insurers or HMOs. Rush institutions have contracts with virtually all of the insurers in the marketplace.

ArcVentures, the for-profit subsidiary of Rush, has a board appointed by

Rush. The board consists of seven people, including two members from the venture-capital community. ArcVentures has developed a number of operating companies over the years. Its contributions to Rush include an operating profit, which accrues to Rush's bottom line, and capital gains realized when it sells any of its operating companies. To date, it has flourished. Two companies were sold, one a national mail-order home pharmacy and the other a home-infusion therapy company. Neither Rush Prudential Health Plans nor ArcVentures is a member of the Rush System for Health. ArcVentures revenues have peaked at approximately $90 million per year, and Rush Prudential's at $450 million. The Rush System for Health is a preferred provider for Rush Prudential Health Plans, and a close working relationship exists.

Governance Structures

Governance of Rush University is the responsibility of the Board of Trustees of Rush-Presbyterian-St. Luke's Medical Center. The board has seen fit to appoint a Board of Overseers for Rush University that currently comprises members of the Board of Trustees of Rush-Presbyterian-St. Luke's Medical Center.

It is important to note that the underlying governance philosophy seeks to integrate Rush with each of its corporately affiliated partners. In the 1970s, Rush experimented with ownership and management of a community hospital in Chicago and decided that the model of ownership and management by the academic health center was less than ideal.

In creating the corporately integrated structures previously described, the intent has been to maintain community stewardship and local management of each of the corporately affiliated partners of the Rush Health System. Maximum autonomy was desired, but the relationship had to be close enough so that the institutions would be recognized by the Federal government as a single business entity and could combine financials. In addition, it was a requirement that the relationships be permanent with no opportunity to withdraw. The bridge board structure accomplishes single business entity status because it is populated by a majority of Rush University trustees and holds the following reserve powers over the corporately integrated affiliate.

1. The power to appoint or ratify the affiliate's Board of Directors.

2. The power to approve the affiliate's strategic plan.

3. The power to approve all debt issuances outside of debt to cover normal operating expenses.

4. The power to approve all affiliations of the corporately integrated partner.

5. The power to assume direct governance control of the affiliate in the circumstance of financial exigency (as defined by failure to meet debt issuance covenants or bankruptcy).

Fortunately the fifth power has never been invoked. In choosing community hospitals with which to integrate, Rush has looked for hospitals that were strong financially, well managed, and enjoyed strong community stewardship. Over the past eight years, several hospitals had to be excluded from selection because of evidence of a less than desirable strength in their financial conditions.

It should be noted that the bridge board does not have authority over medical staff affairs of the corporately integrated institutions. Specifically, it has no authority for medical staff appointment, promotions, or granting privileges. It also does not have authority over medical staff bylaws. Medical staff of the corporate affiliates are not appointed to the faculty of Rush University de facto because of the affiliation. However, those medical staff who participate in the academic programs of the university receive appropriate academic appointments. The president and chief executive officer of RPSLMC serves as the chairman of each of the respective bridge boards. Meetings of the bridge boards are held annually, and to date no substantive differences have arisen at the bridge board level.

Of additional significance, the CEO of each corporately integrated institution is a number of the Management Committee of Rush-Presbyterian-St. Luke's Medical Center, by invitation, not by agreement. This structure allows the CEOs to have intimate knowledge of the workings of the medical center and free access to all of its senior officers. Because of the wide geographic dispersion of the system, the CEOs are not regular attendees at the weekly management committee sessions, but they do feel welcome and included.

Although the various corporately integrated partners have bilateral agreements with Rush that are quite similar in structure, it is interesting that each of them has joined the system for a different reason. In one circumstance, there was the primary desire to include Rush in the corporate name and to develop Rush programs in the institution. In another instance, the primary reason for integrating was access to capital for a new hospital that was subsequently built and is currently in operation. In a third circumstance, the primary reason was for residency and undergraduate medical education programs. Another driving force was access to covered lives through participation in the Rush System for Health.

The largest corporately integrated partner in the Rush System for Health is Illinois Masonic Medical Center, which has an elegant history as a major teaching institution in Chicago. It is also the only affiliate with major tertiary capabilities. The other institutions were primarily community hospitals, and none had residency programs when they entered into their arrangement with Rush-Presbyterian-St. Luke's Medical Center. Today all but three of the member institutions have residency programs or are about to begin such programs under the auspices of Rush.

THE RUSH STRUCTURES: ADVANTAGES AND DISADVANTAGES

What are the advantages and disadvantages of the Rush structures? The Rush model is a very large, diversified system with centralized governance and management structures. This centralization permits rapid decision-making, which is necessary in the Chicago healthcare market. Decisions on new affiliations as additions to the Rush System can be made in a short time frame.

The integration of the hospital and the medical school as a single business unit is advantageous as well. The dean of Rush Medical College is involved in negotiations with potential hospital partners and is, therefore, able, for example, to offer primary care residencies or other programs that may be needed. The tension that often exists between deans and hospital administrators is markedly reduced with this arrangement.

Rush has a very strong Board of Trustees that is extremely supportive of the entrepreneurial activities of the institution. The major leaders of Chicago's industrial sector are members of the board and they appreciate the need for the institution to be able to respond appropriately to the marketplace. The faculty at the downtown academic health center campus comprises both private practice and full-time salaried practitioners. This composition has advantages and disadvantages. One advantage of having private practice physicians is that they are very sensitive to the needs of the market and attuned to changes in the health care marketplace. They are also strong contributors to the clinical academic programs of the institution. The presence of a full-time, salaried faculty ensures the progress of the basic science and clinical missions of the institution and is essential to preserving and enhancing quality development of the academic mission.

The disadvantage of having such a mix of faculty is the challenge it presents for combining the two groups into a cohesive clinical care physician entity capable of single-signature contracting. At Rush, the solution was the creation of a physician hospital organization (PHO), which is jointly owned and governed by the physicians (private practice and salaried) and the hospital. This organization has been remarkably effective in aligning incentives of both private and salaried physicians with the hospital. At the system level, a structure has been put in place that combines all of the PHOs into a single-signature physician contracting organization (the Super-PHO). A system medical services organizations (MSO) has been developed, and is, perhaps, even more important strategically.

One disadvantage of a free-standing academic health center is the lack of nonhealth-related schools as part of the entity. Often, it is important to work with humanities or social science disciplines as well as other disciplines in the sciences. Rush has developed joint relationships with nonhealth-related colleges in Chicago area institutions for specific purposes, often in relation to grant applications.

As a private institution, Rush receives very little public support. The state of Illinois subsidizes the institution for health professions education, and Rush receives approximately $2.2 million a year from the state for this purpose. The entire enterprise must, therefore, face the challenge of basing its operations on its bottom line and shouldering financial responsibility for support of research and education. Currently, the research and education enterprise of Rush University covers its direct costs, but does not cover $11 million of its allocated costs a year. It would be unfair, however, to say that the university costs Rush $11 million annually on its bottom line, because much of the allocated overhead would remain if the university did not exist. The overhead would just have to be allocated across the health care delivery functions of the organization. Since education and research are two of the primary missions of the entire enterprise, this unreimbursed overhead is not seen as a drain on the institution; instead it appears to be quite a bargain. "Without the academic structure of Rush University, the clinical programs would lose their luster, and on a financial basis alone the institution would be less successful, I am sure," says Leo M. Henikoff, MD, president and chief executive officer of Rush-Presbyterian-St. Luke's Medical Center.

In the last two years, Rush has concluded an agreement with Cook County Hospital to be its sole academic affiliate. Many of the educational activities of Rush University both at the undergraduate and graduate levels have been integrated with Cook County Hospital to the benefit of both institutions. Although Cook County Hospital, a public institution, is not a member of the Rush System for Health, it is a very important academic partner of Rush University. In addition, that partnership extends beyond academic activities. Many of the health care programs of the two institutions have been coordinated with some tertiary services being covered by Rush. The Rush Medical College department of emergency medicine is based at Cook County Hospital and under the chairmanship of the director of the department of emergency medicine at Cook County.

CONCLUSION

The Rush System for Health is just leaving its infancy, even though it is twenty-six years old! It is anticipated that the system will evolve as the Chicago market evolves. Member hospitals may find it advantageous to move from the current corporately integrated model into a full asset merger. However, whether this will be viewed collectively as desirable remains to be seen.

The relationship of the Rush System for Health to the Rush Prudential Health Plans could evolve in different ways. If the Rush marketplace remains as fragmented as it is today, then the current strategy of having the system be a provider for all of the insurance companies will continue. However, if Chicago were to become an HMO market with the vast majority of its eight million population in HMOs, Rush Prudential Health Plans could grow with a membership that alone could support the Rush System for Health in terms of covered lives. In such a circumstance, it is likely that unique insurer-provider networks would evolve in the market, and that the Rush Prudential-Rush System for Health partnership would be one of the major entities.

The markets across the country are vastly different from each other and the trends in these marketplaces differ significantly as well. The idea that all markets are moving towards the same end point but are at different points along the way and traveling at different speeds is erroneous. The end points for different markets will not be the same. Fragmented markets such as New York and Chicago will find equilibrium at points far different from markets in California, Minnesota, and Washington state. Academic health centers are also different from each other with different histories and with different constituencies. The Rush model relates only to one institution with one set of traditions and a history in one market. The relevance of this model to other academic health centers will be quite variable.

The Rush mission of health care delivery, education, research, and community service is not going to change. It is an entity with long-term stability ensured by corporate integration and permanent corporate relationships. Its current confederation structure may or may not be adequate to meet the needs of the Chicago market, depending upon the evolution of this market. But the partners are firmly committed to the system, to each other, and to making the proper decisions to meet the needs of the institutions and of the marketplace as the inevitable process of change takes place.

The University of Texas Southwestern Medical Center at Dallas

THE END OF AN ERA OF CROSS-SUBSIDIZATION OF RESEARCH

T HE UNIVERSITY OF TEXAS SOUTHWESTERN Medical Center at Dallas (UT Southwestern) is part of The University of Texas system. From FY 1985 to FY 1995, the total institutional budget at UT Southwestern, which excludes the budget of the teaching hospitals, rose from $182.5 million to $429.6 million. Total research expenditures during this period increased from $46.7 million in 1985 to $94.7 million in 1990 and then to $140.4 million in 1995 (figure 1).

Government research funding, primarily from the National Institutes of Health (NIH), with lesser contributions from the National Science Foundation, the Department of Veterans Affairs, and other Federal agencies, plus a small amount of restricted research funds from the state of Texas, increased from $33.9 to $90.3 million during that period. Private research funding, including money from pharmaceutical company contracts, national organizations such as

This report is based on a presentation by Kern Wildenthal, MD, PhD, president, The University of Texas Southwestern Medical Center at Dallas, at the Task Force on Science Policy of the Association of Academic Health Centers, at its 1996 meeting in Washington.

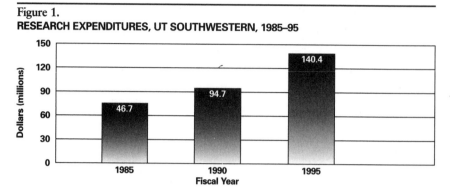

Figure 1.
RESEARCH EXPENDITURES, UT SOUTHWESTERN, 1985–95

the American Heart Association, and local philanthropy increased from $2.8 to $50.1 million.

In 1985, sources of seed dollars to initiate new research programs and to launch young investigators came primarily from general institutional state appropriations (as opposed to funds explicitly appropriated for research). Clinical earnings provided a smaller but significant source of research support. One decade later, however, these sources of cross-subsidization of research had practically vanished, and new sources had to be found.

FUNDING SOURCES
State Appropriations

Each institution within the University of Texas system gets a separate budget from the state legislature. State support per enrolled medical student is almost equal among the schools. There are a few extra dollars for special items, such as research at UT Southwestern, outreach programs for rural medicine at Texas Tech University, and development of health programs along the Mexican border at San Antonio, but special items account for less than 10 percent of total appropriations.

Currently, the state appropriation is sufficient to cover the core costs of medical student education, but the costs of resident training, charity care, and research are not covered to a significant extent by the state. UT Southwestern has to find other funds to subsidize these areas.

From the mid-1960s to the mid-1980s, general state appropriations grew rapidly and were sufficient not only to fund undergraduate education, but also to provide a major means for helping underwrite research, charity care, and the education of medical residents. However, the Texas recession of 1985–86 led to a 13 percent across-the-board reduction of state funds to all institutions of higher education, and subsequent appropriations have failed to keep up with inflation. The result has been the loss of the ability to maintain cross-subsidization of graduate medical education, charity care, and research activities from general state appropriations.

Texas has a competitive grant program of $30 million a year for scientific research projects that are peer-reviewed by out-of-state reviewers. This amount has not grown over the past decade, which means that, when adjusted for inflation, it has fallen (figure 2). Approximately $6 million of that funding goes to the medical schools, with UT Southwestern getting approximately $2 million per year. Another $34 million of state research funding comes to UT Southwestern from special line items that the institution has received from the legislature to support specific projects. These special items, which, at the Federal level, would be considered pork and detrimental to quality-based distribution of funding, have been the only way to provide increased funds for research at the state level.

In summary, state appropriations for UT Southwestern totaled about $62.5 million in 1985; they dropped drastically through 1987, and began to creep back up with inflation, reaching $66 million by 1990. In 1995, at $75.7 million, they were well below 1985 levels when corrected for inflation. The 1995 state appropriation was adequate to support the core undergraduate education mission, but inadequate to subsidize residency education, charity care, and research.

Clinical Income and the Practice Plan

From the 1960s through 1985, when increases in state funds fueled UT

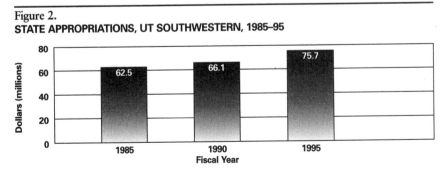

Figure 2.
STATE APPROPRIATIONS, UT SOUTHWESTERN, 1985–95

Figure 3.
PRACTICE PLAN INCOME, UT SOUTHWESTERN, 1985–95

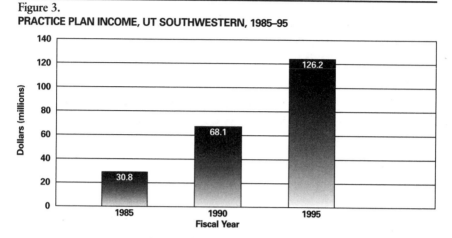

Southwestern's growth, the institution generated relatively little clinical earnings. The campus hospital was the county charity hospital, and there was no inpatient or outpatient capacity for referred and private patients. Texas had miserable Medicaid reimbursement patterns. Therefore, the gross income from clinical earnings that could be used to cross-subsidize other activities was fairly small.

Except for Galveston, the medical schools in Texas (Dallas, San Antonio, Houston, Texas Tech, Texas A&M, and the University of North Texas Osteopathic School) cannot by law own or operate a hospital facility, although they can and do own and operate outpatient facilities. In the 1980s, UT Southwestern built a private referral outpatient facility and, at the institution's request, philanthropists in the community formed a 501(c)(3) corporation to build and operate a university hospital on the campus. The new hospital's mission was to provide a university referral and teaching facility for the faculty of UT Southwestern. Built for 150 beds, there are now 120 staffed beds at the university hospital and the occupancy rate is 75 percent. The hospital lost money during its early years in operation, but has maintained a positive $1–2 million bottom line in recent years. Like other institutions, UT Southwestern and its hospital partners think it would be desirable in the future to affiliate formally with one or more health care systems to remain viable.

It was hoped that provision of facilities for an expanded faculty practice would allow a major expansion of clinical earnings through the faculty practice plan, and thereby provide a means to cross-subsidize other activities as state funds fell. And, indeed, UT Southwestern has succeeded in increasing its total clinical earnings dramatically over the last 10 years; they rose from $30.9 million in 1985 to $68.1 million in 1990 to $126.2 million in 1995 (figure 3).

Dean's Tax

However, gross numbers can be misleading. In 1985, the dean's tax totaled less than $8 million. Although this figure was fairly small, the generosity of state funding, plus the reasonably high reimbursement rates received from paying patents, resulted in a situation where there was relatively little need to use the dean's fund to support core functions and more than $3 million could be applied to subsidizing research. In 1995, the dean's tax grossed over $30 million, which theoretically might have been used to help underwrite research and other activities. However, in 1995, the actual ability of the dean's tax to support research was zero—state underwriting of clinical functions had disappeared and reduced reimbursement rates had caused the "profit" from clinical earnings to fall to the point that any significant capacity to cross-subsidize research had been lost.

It should be noted that the dean's fund is defined differently by different people. Faculty members say that it is a 25 percent tax on the gross collections. The dean of medicine says that the dean's fund is now essentially zero because it is used entirely to support the costs of the clinical operation and provides nothing extra for the dean to use to cross-subsidize other activities. From this 25 percent tax, UT Southwestern pays all the costs of operating the clinic, billing and collecting, marketing, and clinical administration. Thus, the 25 percent dean's tax is now devoted to salaries and expenses for operating the clinical infrastructure. About $2 million a year is used for expanding the clinical programs, including allocations for recruiting new clinicians, especially primary care providers.

Each department still has a small amount of its 75 percent that it can use to underwrite clinical investigation. This is a difficult area to cost-account. Department chairpersons point out convincingly that, even though there has been a fourfold increase in gross revenues over the last 10 years, the amount of discretionary funds of the departments, like the dean's fund, has fallen precipitously. In 1985, a fairly large portion of the departmental 75 percent could be used to support the research of new faculty, beyond those allocations received from the dean's fund, but in 1995 almost all the income was required for paying clinicians' salaries and clinical expenses.

In summary, from 1985 to 1995, the institution lost almost all of its capacity to subsidize research from clinical profits. The practice plan's total income growth is impressive but, in fact, the increase is due to increased patient volumes with reduced margins, and the gross income is used to pay the costs of providing care. For the future, UT Southwestern's basic assumption is that the practice plan will grow, but so will the costs of providing services. Therefore, the practice plan cannot be expected to become a major source for underwriting other activities, such as research.

OTHER OPTIONS FOR
CROSS-SUBSIDIZATION

State funds are no longer a source of cross-subsidization. Even though practice plan earnings are increasing in absolute dollars, they are decreasing in terms of profits that can be used for cross-subsidization. What are the alternative sources?

Recovering the Cost of Charity Care

In 1985, UT Southwestern recognized that both a significant amount of state dollars and a major fraction of practice plan earnings were being used to underwrite faculty time to care for charity patients. The institution tried strenuously to persuade the state legislature that faculty time devoted to caring for charity patients was an important state function, which the state should recognize in its appropriations, but the response from the state was negative. In fact, in 1987, the Texas legislature attached a rider to the appropriations bill explicitly stating that the cost of nonmedical charity care was a county responsibility, not the state's. The rider instructed the medical schools to contract with county hospitals to recover the costs of charity care. Except for the University of Texas Medical Branch at Galveston, which owns its own hospital, the state no longer appropriates funds for charity care at its medical schools.

With regard to Dallas County, UT Southwestern took the position that, because of decreasing state funds, the medical school could not continue to provide the current level of faculty services at the county's Parkland Memorial Hospital unless the county provided more funding for faculty salaries. (To illus-

Figure 4.
CONTRACT WITH PARKLAND MEMORIAL HOSPITAL FOR INDIGENT CARE, 1985–95

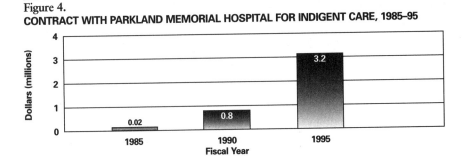

trate the magnitude of the problem, the 1995 unbilled charges for physician services to non-Medicare and non-Medicaid-covered charity patients were over $130 million.) In view of the legislature's mandate, UT Southwestern focused its efforts on persuading the Dallas community that state law required the county to pay for faculty physician services for charity patients.

Fortunately, with the help of a supportive hospital administration (and the necessity of withdrawing services if funds were not forthcoming), UT Southwestern was able to receive increased support from the county (figure 4). In 1995, the institution received $29.2 million for the $130 million worth of services that were provided. Although not an enormous rate of return, it is considerably better than the $2.8 million the institution had received in 1985. This $26.4 million increase in UT Southwestern's annual budget has been of vital importance in preserving the integrity of the institution.

Royalty Income

Like other academic health centers, UT Southwestern has tried over the last ten years to maximize income that could be used to support research through technology transfer agreements and royalties. The institution's success in this regard has been dramatic, with income rising from $20,000 a year in 1985 to $800,000 in 1990 to $3.2 million in 1995 (figure 5).

Once again, however, the gross numbers do not tell the full story. The institution's policy is to share licensing and patent income fifty-fifty with the inventor. The institution's share is then divided between the department or laboratory that generated the research and an unrestricted institutional research fund. Thus far, the research fund share has been required to support the operations of the

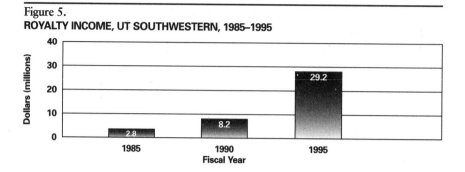

Figure 5.
ROYALTY INCOME, UT SOUTHWESTERN, 1985–1995

technology office. Expenses incurred on behalf of a particular patent or contract are taken from the income produced by that patent or contract. But funds to underwrite the expenses of those patents that never produce any revenue have to be subsidized from the institution's 25 percent share in the research fund. Thus, funds to subsidize generic research have not yet been realized, although the successful laboratories have realized money to subsidize their own research.

The bulk of the technology transfer income results from the work of a few laboratories. In fact, one laboratory accounts for more than 60 percent of the funds, a second laboratory accounts for another 20 percent, and forty laboratories account for the remaining 20 percent. Income from royalties is useful, but it has not created a way to cross-subsidize research beyond providing funds for the generating laboratories.

Private Gift Support

The most successful strategy for generating funds for supporting clinical and basic research at UT Southwestern has been to seek gifts from private donors. Total philanthropic support in 1985 was $10.7 million, of which less than $2 million came from the community (figure 6). The primary sources of philanthropic funds at that time were national granting agencies, such as the American Heart Association and the American Cancer Society. In 1990, private gift support had risen to $30.7 million and, by 1995, total donations were $49.2 million, with over $30 million coming from the community. This figure includes support for all institutional purposes (research, scholarships, and clinical programs); however, the majority goes for research, which has proven to be the activity that is, by far, the most appealing for donors.

In most medical schools, alumni are only occasionally a major source of philanthropic gifts. Thus, unlike most universities, medical schools rarely focus their major fund-raising efforts on alumni. Instead, the primary source of most gifts to medical centers is grateful patients. Unlike most medical centers, however, UT Southwestern has historically provided care almost exclusively for charity patients. Grateful patients have, therefore, been responsible for only a small fraction of the institution's philanthropic funds. In the future, however, it is anticipated that the percentage of support coming from grateful patients will increase along with the expanding referral care base. This is one potential benefit from the institution's investment in increasing clinical services, even if clinical "profits" are small.

Over the past decade, however, with a relative dearth of wealthy patients, it has been necessary to attract a different philanthropic population. UT Southwestern, therefore, has focused its efforts on involving local foundations, businesses, and individuals whose primary motives for giving are more generic: general altruism, the desire to conquer disease, and civic pride. UT Southwestern has benefited from being the only medical school in Dallas; it is an even greater benefit to be the only university program in Dallas that is regarded as world class. Accordingly, the institution has devoted considerable attention to building up its image in the community and, for the past decade, has focused its development strategy on local private philanthropy based largely on civic pride.

In 1985, the development office consisted of one secretary who wrote and typed letters of appreciation for any gifts that happened to arrive. In 1986, a

Figure 6.
PRIVATE GIFTS, UT SOUTHWESTERN, 1985–95

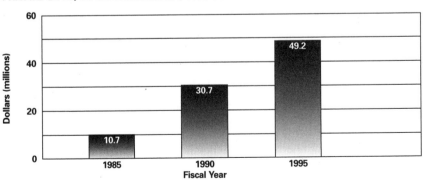

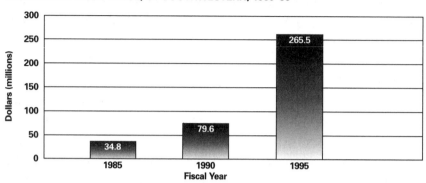

Figure 7.
ENDOWMENT BOOK VALUE, UT SOUTHWESTERN, 1985–95

small professional development office was created and a public awareness effort was initiated. By 1995, the total development budget had grown to $600,000. Development costs are thus less than 2 percent of gift income.

Fund-raising efforts at UT Southwestern have been concentrated on major gifts. More than 75 percent of local philanthropic funds come from donors who give $1 million or more. For further growth, it will be necessary to expand the donor base and appeal to a broader segment of the population. Dallas is growing rapidly, and the new wealth is in the suburbs. A development effort with one president and two development officers cannot adequately cover the entire geographic area and its population. UT Southwestern plans to enlarge the development office in an effort to expand its donor base throughout the metropolitan area, in addition to maintaining the core philanthropic base in central Dallas that has been built over the past decade.

The institution attempts to steer most of its philanthropic dollars into endowments. This results in a temporary postponement of institutional growth and improvement, but produces an important element of future stability. From its establishment in 1943, to 1985, UT Southwestern's endowments had grown to only $35 million; by 1990, however, the endowment book value had more than doubled to $80 million and, by 1995, endowments totaled $265 million (figure 7). In comparison with many medical schools, the school's endowment is still relatively small, but the rate at which the endowment is increasing and UT Southwestern's annual receipts from fund-raising are larger than most.

One problem that has been brought about by the successful pursuit of gifts for research, is that most donors (including agencies such as the American Cancer Society and the American Heart Association) will not pay full overhead costs. The need to identify sources of funding to cover the indirect costs of research that accompany expenditures fueled by donors remains to be addressed.

CONCLUSION

Grants from NIH and other national agencies that use peer review account for the majority of research funds received by UT Southwestern, but these cannot be relied on to provide start-up funds for innovative research projects or for launching the research efforts of new faculty members. The traditional sources of cross-subsidization of research—state appropriations and profits from clinical practice—have become inadequate over the past decade, and it is not likely that this trend will be reversed. State funds, corrected for inflation, are also decreasing and no longer provide a significant source of funds for underwriting research, charity care, or graduate medical education. The practice plan has increased fourfold over the past decade and now constitutes a much larger fraction of the institutional budget: but, paradoxically, it contributes less toward underwriting research and other activities because of a reduced profit margin.

UT Southwestern's strategy for dealing with the problem of finding funds to support research has been to pursue three avenues:

1. A successful effort has been made to persuade the county government to cover more of the costs of physician services for charity patients so that practice plan income is not required for that purpose to an overwhelming extent; this allows the remaining clinical profits of the departments, small though they be, to be available, in part, for cross-subsidizing research.

2. A vigorous technology transfer program has been moderately successful, although the program generates significant funds for only a few laboratories.

3. Most important, a concerted effort to increase charitable contributions yielded a fifteenfold increase in local philanthropic support for research between 1985 and 1995. Total charitable donations have risen to approximately $50 million a year. Philanthropic support of research appears to be the best source of funds to compensate for the loss of cross-subsidization capability from state appropriations and clinical profits.

Tulane University and Columbia/HCA

SELLING A UNIVERSITY HOSPITAL TO A FOR-PROFIT SYSTEM

THE PROCESS THAT LED TO THE SALE OF TULANE University Hospital, which was wholly owned by the university, started in early 1992. The hospital, a 300-bed facility with an adjoining fourth-floor ambulatory care center, was the clinical service component of the Tulane University Medical Center.

Tulane has a two-tier governing system. The board of administrators is the fiduciary body for the university, of which the medical center is a part, and a corporate entity of the university. The board of governors of the medical center does not have separate corporate responsibility, except as delegated by the board of administrators. However, the board of administrators does delegate a substantial portion of responsibility for the medical center to the board of governors.

MERGER AND OTHER OPTIONS

Both boards had been discussing the future of the hospital as a result of the changing economic picture. They were concerned with new legislative initia-

This report was prepared by John C. LaRosa, MD, chancellor of the Tulane University Medical Center. It is based on presentations by Dr. Eamon Kelly, former president of Tulane University, and Dr. LaRosa at the Forum on University Relations of the Association of Academic Health Centers in Washington, DC, in 1996.

tives as well as with economic issues and the Tulane health care marketplace. Discussions became formal in January 1993 when a joint board committee was established to oversee staff studies related to the future of the university and the impact of legislation and market forces on the hospital and the medical center.

This newly formed joint committee was composed of the chairman of the board of administrators, the chairman of the board of governors, the president of the university, and the chancellor of the medical center. In addition, a separate task force, made up of representatives of the faculty and staff of the medical center, focused on the following five areas: operations, medical education (undergraduate and graduate), research, health care delivery, and the faculty practice plan.

The importance of the joint board committee and the task force cannot be understated. The governing boards and the faculty were deeply involved very early in the process, which facilitated many later activities. The report of the joint board committee was released in September 1993, and was quite extensive, addressing the financial picture and the options for the future.

The worst case scenario in the financial section of the report predicted that the hospital would move from a $30 million surplus to an $18 million deficit in a period of 2–3 years. The university president faced the possibility of creating deficits of $15–20 million a year in a short period of time.

The deliberations of the board and faculty led to the consideration of four options. One option was to develop a Tulane network, but this idea did not appear feasible because of the levels of capital infusion that would be required. A second option was to merge with another institution. This idea was based on the belief that any viable strategy would require a market share of 20 percent of beds in the future. The third option was to sell health care delivery assets (the hospital). The fourth option was to become a provider of specialized services and pin survival on developing services that were not available elsewhere. The faculty reviewed these studies and recommended the merger option; their second choice was the sale of the hospital assets.

As a result of this recommendation, negotiations for a possible merger with Ochsner Clinic began in January 1994. After five months, however, it was clear that such a partnership was not going to work. In May or June (by which time the failed negotiations had become public knowledge), the university was approached by Columbia Health Care about a possible venture that would include both Tulane and Louisiana State University (LSU). Tulane expressed a willingness to meet with the principals of Columbia/HCA. LSU declined.

In the initial discussion, Tulane presented its requirements, which included: (1) the development of a network that had a market share of at least 20 percent and that generated patients for both tertiary care and research; (2) joint governance and protection of medical education and research; and (3) the potential to receive substantial cash transactions. Columbia representatives quickly agreed to these broad requirements.

In June 1994, the president, the board of administrators, and the board of governors formed a negotiating group. The group, whose members changed from time to time, had 12 to 14 people and included members from both boards, staff, and faculty representatives from the medical school. The three faculty representatives were the elected head of the faculty plan, the chief of staff of the hospital, and the chair of the clinical science council (the clinical chairpersons group). These three were key members of the negotiating team.

Negotiations began in June 1994 and, by September 1994, a letter of intent was approved by the joint boards. Between September 1994 and January 1995, this highly detailed letter of intent became a negotiated arrangement. In January 1995, the boards approved the deal. They also created, at the president's suggestion, an allocation committee to determine the process by which the cash from the transaction would be appropriated within the university. This avoided an internal struggle over the distribution of the proceeds, an issue neither the board nor the university senate could handle. A three-person committee was formed, comprising a member of the board of administrators, a member of the Board of Governors, and a third individual who was not a member of either board. The committee was given final executive authority to allocate the assets. The faculty and boards were overwhelmingly in favor of the transaction.

The public signing took place on March 31, 1995. Many legal and financial experts have commented on the extremely complex nature of this transaction. The technical aspects of the transaction made it very complicated, specifically, the university had to tender all of its existing tax-exempt bonds, and other sets of bonds had to be repurchased. (Certain established trusts cannot sell their bonds, which became a problem.) Although the bond component was the most complicated part of the deal, the overall amount of documentation required was enormous.

The goal of the sale of Tulane University Hospital was to better position the medical center in the New Orleans health care marketplace, which is currently very immature in terms of managed care with only 15–20 percent penetration. At the time the discussions started, there was only 10 percent penetration.

GOVERNANCE ISSUES

Faculty involvement in the process was critical. The initial plan was to have the dean of medicine represent the faculty. Upon reflection, it was decided to expand the group to include those members of the faculty who had been elected to their given administrative post. They included the chief of staff of the hospital, the chairman of the clinical departmental group, and the medical directors of the faculty practice plan. These people communicated directly with the faculty, which made an enormous difference in the faculty's overwhelming acceptance of the proposal.

A limited liability company, named University Health Systems, Ltd., was formed with 20 percent of the equity owned by Tulane and 80 percent by Columbia. Tulane's liability is limited to its investment in University Health Systems, Ltd., and the university's nonprofit tax status is maintained. No taxes are collected on whatever profits are distributed to the university. The university, however, plays a substantial role in the governance of the new company.

The governing board of the company has 10 members and is distinct from the medical center's board of governors. The latter oversees the schools, the research centers, and the practice plan, but has no authority in hospital governance. The new hospital board has five members from Columbia and five members from Tulane, with the chair named by Tulane. All major decisions must be approved by a majority of both Columbia and Tulane board members. Thus, three of the five Columbia members and three of the five Tulane members have to approve any major decisions for the company. Decisions requiring majority approval include hiring or firing the hospital CEO; transfer, creation, or deletion of any hospital service; modification of academic support; or the purchase of any other teaching hospital within a 75-mile radius.

STAFFING

All house staff programs are maintained at their current size with the important caveat that any reductions in graduate medical education support by Medicare and Medicaid are passed through. Even so, this will involve negotiations in that a resident (even nonreimbursed) may be the most cost-effective means of providing hospital coverage.

The faculty has no restrictions in terms of applying for privileges at other hospitals. Faculty members may (and do) hold appointments in a number of hospitals around the city.

CAPITALIZATION AND PRACTICE PLAN

The capitalization of the new company is straightforward. Columbia contributed $132 million in assets, and Tulane contributed $33 million. The clinical faculty (but not the practice plan) was transferred to Columbia along with the hospital. As a result, the practice plan experienced a dramatic reduction in overhead, from about 45 percent to 27 percent. The hospital/clinic, however, now charges a separate facility fee. While this change has proved positive for the practice plan in one sense, it has also led to the patients complaining about receiving two bills.

Annual support, including house debt support and support for medical service directors who also have educational roles in the hospital as faculty, is approximately $22 million. In addition, Columbia agreed to a line of credit to fund a five-year, $75 million capital improvement plan for the hospital. Another $75 million credit has been committed to developing clinical centers of excellence. To service this debt, the continued profitable operation of the hospital is required.

CENTERS OF EXCELLENCE

Columbia agreed to support several approved centers of clinical excellence in the hospital and clinic. Business plans for a cancer center and sports medicine center have been agreed on, and several others are in the works. This has proved an interesting educational process for both parties. The business plans are rigorous and realistic (not always the case in academic planning), but also include allowances for teaching and research.

Columbia has also recognized, in principle, that if Tulane is going to continue to grow as an academic center and become a cutting-edge institution, investments must be made in areas where the payoff may not be immediate. Such centers will help establish a reputation for the institution, but may not be income producers for some time. Precisely how the introduction of centers of excellence will be implemented remains to be seen.

NETWORK DEVELOPMENT

In the New Orleans area, Columbia is forming a regional network of hospitals, ambulatory facilities, and practices, with Tulane as the academic center. During the negotiations, the medical center independently formed a committee to consider the components of both an ideal service network and an ideal teaching network in the region. The service network plans have formed the basis for ongoing discussions and planning with Columbia. The academic network has some components common to the service network, as well as some that are independent. As a result, there will be an overlap of Tulane's service network, Tulane's academic network, and Columbia's service networks in the state and region.

Network development is moving forward as a result of regular meetings between Tulane and local, regional, and state officials from Columbia. Broadly speaking, the network will be structured on individual physician-hospital organizations, with an overarching medical services organization. In practice, the boundaries of the network have grown to include a larger area of the state than initially envisioned. Some referral services have already been established at Tulane. For example, Tulane is the referral center for Louisiana and Texas for organ and bone marrow transplants. Columbia is currently negotiating with a number of large practices, some of which are primary care and some subspecialty oriented.

Columbia has been very flexible about expectations for financial performance, but it is nevertheless very disciplined. Targets are expected to be met and progress is examined carefully and frequently.

IMPACT OF THE MERGER

A question often asked of Tulane (although perhaps not properly directed) is: What does Columbia get out of the merger deal? Clearly, it has acquired a strong relationship with a tertiary care research center with positive marketing potential. Also, Columbia is in the position to develop a model for how private sector medicine can contribute to the survival of academic institutions.

The arrangement is still too new to draw definitive conclusions about the impact on Tulane. Thus far, however, the impact has been positive, as seen by the following developments:

- Income has stabilized.
- New support for capital and centers of excellence has been identified.
- Faculty anxiety has been reduced and there is a general sense of optimism.
- Plans for a family practice program, underwritten by Columbia, are underway.
- A health policy research institute, also underwritten by Columbia, is firmly established.
- A strategic plan, including the Columbia relationship, has been completed and is being implemented.

Wake Forest University/Bowman Gray School of Medicine

EXPLORING THE FUTURE ORGANIZATION OF ACADEMIC HEALTH CENTERS

THE WAKE FOREST UNIVERSITY ACADEMIC HEALTH center in Winston-Salem, North Carolina, comprises a school of medicine and four other health professions programs (dentistry, public health sciences, allied health, and the Graduate School of Arts and Sciences of Wake Forest University), two major, affiliated teaching hospitals with more than 1,750 beds, and a research enterprise that receives more than $70 million in direct grants annually. Full-time enrollment in the health professions schools was 1,168 in 1996, and 1,100 other students received their clinical experience in nursing and allied professions at the medical center. The academic health center campus, known as the Hawthorne campus, is four and a half miles from the main university campus, also located in Winston-Salem.

This report is based on a presentation by Richard Janeway, MD, then executive vice president for health affairs at Wake Forest University and chief executive officer of Bowman Gray School of Medicine, at the Association of Academic Health Centers' symposium on The Future of Academic Health Centers in 1996 in Chicago. Since this report, Wake Forest University/Bowman Gray School of Medicine has been renamed Wake Forest University School of Medicine.

Wake Forest is one of four academic health centers in the state. The Wake Forest medical school, founded in 1902, was originally a two-year school. In 1939, Bowman Gray, chairman of the board of the Reynolds Tobacco Company, bequeathed almost $600,000 to any one of North Carolina's two-year medical schools that would relocate to Winston-Salem, become a four-year school, and take North Carolina Baptist Hospital as its hospital partner. The School of Medicine, renamed the School of Medical Sciences, accepted the offer, agreed to the terms of the will, and moved from Wake County to Winston-Salem in 1941. At that time, it was renamed the Bowman Gray School of Medicine of Wake Forest College in recognition of the benefactor who made the expansion possible.

In 1946, the trustees of Wake Forest College and the Baptist State Convention of North Carolina accepted a proposal by the Z. Smith Reynolds Foundation to relocate the Wake Forest College within Winston-Salem. In 1956, the college moved all operations to the Southeastern Baptist Theological Seminary, leaving the 122-year-old campus in the town of Wake Forest. The decade that followed was the college's most expansive and, in 1967, its increased size and scope was recognized by the change in name to Wake Forest University (WFU).

Today, enrollment in the university stands at more than 5,000. Governance remains in the hands of the board of trustees, and development for each of the five schools of the university is assisted by the board of visitors for the undergraduate college and graduate school, the school of medicine, the school of law, and the graduate school of management.

Winston-Salem is a small community with a population of 161,000. Forsyth County has a population of 276,000. The total primary service area for the medical center has a population of about three million and consists of nineteen counties in northwestern North Carolina and six counties in southwestern Virginia. The secondary service area for the university extends to Guilford County in the east and Mecklenberg County in the south, and to Tennessee in the west. The medical center is developing a regional, integrated delivery system throughout its primary service area, and plans to extend service throughout North Carolina via a variety of cooperative agreements.

Figure 1.
ORGANIZATION AND GOVERNANCE STRUCTURE, MEDICAL CENTER, BOWMAN GRAY SCHOOL OF MEDICINE AND NORTH CAROLINA BAPTIST HOSPITAL

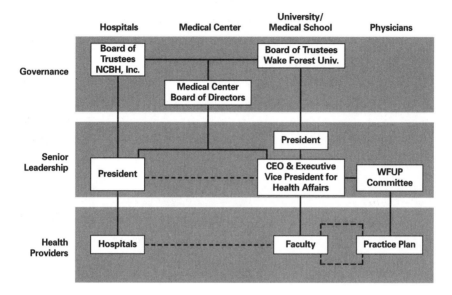

ORGANIZATION AND GOVERNANCE

The governance structure of the university provides a great deal of flexibility in medical school decision-making. The work of the medical school is divided among twenty-eight departments. The control of the medical school is vested in the board of trustees of Wake Forest University. Although part of the university, the medical school operates under an appendix of the university bylaws that cedes all of the organizational and financial affairs of the school of medicine to the executive vice president for health affairs/chief executive officer of the Bowman Gray School of Medicine. The executive vice president reports to the president of the university (figure 1).

Many of the functions within the medical center have been centralized. The medical center has its own board of directors, equally represented from the boards of trustees of the university and the North Carolina Baptist Hospital, which oversees all centralized functions (e.g., information services, public relations, strategic planning, and development).

Table 1.

BOWMAN GRAY SCHOOL OF MEDICINE CLINICAL SERVICES BUDGETS, 1995–97

Sources:	Budget 1995–96	Actual Spent 1995–96	Approved Budget 1996–97
WFUP	$119,895	$127,524	$134,765
Professional Services – NCBH	12,348	13,596	13,151
Dialysis	20,458	20,638	21,370
Other	9,114	7,546	9,951
Total	161,815	169,304	179,237
Uses:			
Education/Research/Patient Care	134,402	137,749	149,485
Other	4,149	5,411	5,750
Transfers			
Faculty Pledge	4,550	4,533	4,690
R&D	16,152	15,815	16,454
Other	2,562	4,256	2,858
Total	161,815	167,765	179,237
Contributions to Reserves	0	1,540	0

BUDGET

Gross revenues for the medical center for 1996 were approximately $940 million. The net revenue for North Carolina Baptist Hospitals, Inc., was approximately $410 million; for the Bowman Gray School of Medicine of Wake Forest, it was $301 million. Of that $301 million, $167 million was from clinical revenues that included $17.2 million in payments for professional services from hospitals, $74 million in research and "demonstration program" support, and about $51–52 million in unrestricted income from tuition, interest, endowment income, and indirect cost reimbursement (overhead) from research programs.

The breakdown of the revenue sources for the $179.2 million budgeted for 1996–97 is as follows: $134.8 million of professional service revenues from Wake Forest University Physicians (the integrated, multidisciplinary group practice); $13.2 million from professional services rendered to the North Carolina Baptist Hospital and other affiliates; $21.4 million from kidney dialysis operations in six different locations in North Carolina; and $9.7 million from other sources (table 1). In addition, $16.5 million in "foregone professional income" is used to support departmental research and development. This amount, which represents the cross-subsidy of the academic and research element of the medical school by the clinical faculty, is in addition to the faculty pledge of 5.15 percent of their net revenues to the dean's office ($4.7 million), which also supports academic endeavors, and a 2 percent charge on end-of-year balances of departmental research and development funds ($1.8 million). Direct clinical "subsidy" of academic pursuits is at least $23 million per year. Interest on invested research and development fund balances ($8 million) brings direct and indirect support to $31 million per year.

THE HOSPITAL AND FACULTY PRACTICE

The North Carolina Baptist Hospital (NCBH), with 806 licensed beds, is the primary affiliated teaching hospital of the university and one of the largest in the region and the country. In 1996, it had 24,315 inpatient visits, which was 2.4 percent higher than in 1994–95. Currently, inpatient admissions are running 8 percent over budget for the 1996 academic year, which belies the conventional wisdom that tertiary and quaternary medical centers of necessity suffer under managed care. Patient days have decreased overall as a result of efficiencies in hospital operations. The average length of stay was reduced by 1.3 days in the past two years. There were 516,419 ambulatory visits in 1995; visits increased by 7 percent in 1996 to 552,475.

Bowman Gray operates the Reynolds Health Center for the county, where there were an additional 56,000 patient encounters in 1995–96, many for the treatment of indigent patients. The clinic is a very important part of Wake Forest's teaching program in the ambulatory arena. The total clinical enterprise revenue for 1996 was about $580 million. The Baptist Hospital services 4,952 Medicaid and 9,911 Medicare patients and writes off about $200 million annually in free care, contractual adjustments, and bad debts. All obstetrical services are conducted at the community affiliate, Forsyth Memorial Hospital (924 beds), which has about 6,000 deliveries annually.

North Carolina is slightly behind the rest of the country with regard to managed care penetration, which statewide was about 8.7 percent in 1994 as compared to 21.1 percent nationwide (figure 2). In 1996, approximately 11 percent of the state population were in managed care; nationally, the average was

Figure 2.
HMO PENETRATION IN NORTH CAROLINA, 1989–94

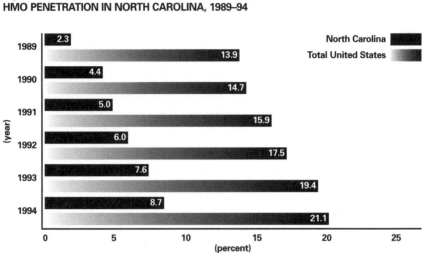

Sources: Managed Care Digest, HMO Edition 1992–94, Maron Merrell Dow; Managed Care Digest Series, HMO-PPO Digest 1995, Hoechst-Maron-Roussel.

21 percent. Winston-Salem/Forsyth County, however, has about 57 percent of the employed population (and their dependents) enrolled in some type of managed care organization, the majority of which are controlled by the Partners National Health Care Corporation, which, until recently, was 55 percent owned by community physicians.

The university does not own its principal teaching hospital, but the full-time university faculty essentially comprise the hospital staff, with the exception of pediatrics. The part-time faculty have admitting privileges. Until two years ago, the hospital was a totally closed-staff hospital, meaning that a staff member had to first be appointed to the faculty before he or she received privileges at the hospital. Indeed, the university, not the hospital, determines who has admitting privileges to the hospital. The hospital trustees determine the clinical privileges a physician can receive.

Bowman Gray has a totally integrated faculty practice governed by an advisory committee that reports to the executive vice president for health affairs. With the encouragement of the Bowman Gray administration, WFUP is moving toward a multidisciplinary group practice that will become more self-governing, with the majority of the council elected by the MD faculty of the clinical departments. The leadership of the council must be approved by the executive vice president for health affairs. Bowman Gray has 403 full-time physicians involved in its clinical practice, which is totally integrated within the medical center structure. The new council will supervise overall plans and incentive structures that will govern the multidisciplinary group practice. All support functions of the medical center such as billing, collections, and appointment scheduling, in addition to those mentioned earlier, will eventually come under singular guidance and control.

RELATIONSHIP WITH COMMUNITY PRACTITIONERS

Many experts believe that academic health centers should be at a competitive advantage in relation to the practicing physician community. Wake Forest decided in the 1960s not to compete with the physicians practicing in the community. Consequently, the medical center did not compete locally in either primary or most secondary care. (The medical school graduated 52 percent of specialists practicing in the county.) As a consequence of this posture, Bowman Gray has only a 24 percent market share in Forsyth County, while the community physicians hold a 76 percent market share. In the twenty-six counties surrounding Forsyth, the opposite is true; Wake Forest has a 76 percent share of the market. However, the local hospital and physician organization is actively moving to increase its presence in the Wake Forest referral area through the establishment of satellite practices and by marketing the Partners HMO.

TENURE

Tenure arrangements and faculty teaching time will have to be addressed in every medical school in the United States. In the 1980s, the Bowman Gray School of Medicine modified tenure. Five years is the time allowed for appointment. At the end of five years, all faculty members are evaluated and peer reviewed. If the review is not positive, there is a two-year guaranteed remediation process to which the university is obligated. If, after two years, the evaluation is still not positive, the faculty member is terminated. All university appeals and grievance policies and procedures have been retained and assiduously applied. The process has been tested and upheld by actions brought through the Equal Employment Opportunity Commission.

STRATEGIES FOR THE FUTURE

Recognizing that health care reform and the growth of managed care would transform the delivery of health care in North Carolina, the Bowman Gray medical center created a task force in 1992 to reassess the market and evaluate future strategies for the university. The task force recommended that the academic health center develop an integrated delivery system, an insurance product, primary care capability, and an advanced information system. For an academic institution, Wake Forest moved quite rapidly to act on these recommendations. By December 1993, the university had completed a feasibility study for its insurance product. In February 1994, the university created an incorporated for-profit HMO entity, QualChoice of North Carolina, Inc., which was licensed in North Carolina in September 1994. In December 1994, two companies were created, a 501(c)(3) physician acquisition and affiliation foundation model, called Aegis Family Health Centers, and a for-profit management service organization, called Management Directions of North Carolina, which was a limited liability corporation.

The Integrated Delivery System Environment

In 1986, Winston-Salem community specialists and the Forsyth Memorial Hospital, a privatized county hospital operating as Carolina Medicorp, Inc. (CMI), went into partnership with Aetna Life Insurance Company, creating an HMO called Partners National Health Plans of North Carolina. In 1987, enrollment was 3,700. By the end of 1996, approximately 120,000 people were enrolled in the plan, now wholly owned by CMI, which bought out the physicians in a transaction valued at $84 million in early 1996.

QualChoice of North Carolina

For its insurance product, Wake Forest University and North Carolina Baptist Hospital in 1994 established QualChoice of North Carolina, Inc., which adopted the Novalis Model Triple Option Point of Service Plan. Many people consider Novalis to be a superb plan for academic health centers because the patient has a great deal of freedom of choice in physician selection at each encounter. Financial decisions also rest with the patient. The board of trustees approved the plan, and, in February 1994, QualChoice was incorporated as a

Figure 3.
CLIENTS OF MANAGEMENT DIRECTIONS OF NORTH CAROLINA

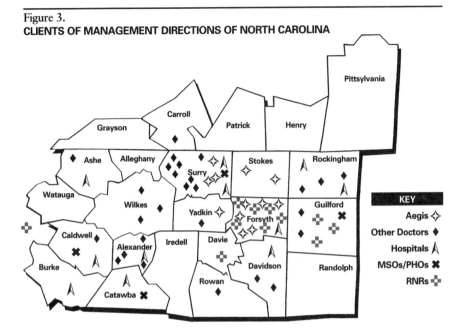

for-profit HMO. However, QualChoice was launched only after much turmoil. Primary care and specialist physicians in the community boycotted the HMO, and the boycott was broken only by threat of legal action. This turmoil precipitated an aggressive battle for the acquisition of physicians. CMI now "owns" 49 percent of all the private practice internists and family practitioners in Forsyth County and 67 percent of the pediatricians. The medical center "owns" almost all the remaining private practices in the same specialties.

As of December 31, 1995, the enrollment in QualChoice was approximately 30,000. Enrollment was expected to increase beyond 50,000 by the end of December 1996. The network has been expanded to 950 physicians throughout the Wake Forest referral area; 55 percent are primary care physicians. Most of the 45 percent who are specialists work within the medical center, but there are specialty providers in all the communities served. There are thirteen practice sites for the Aegis Family Health Centers, which are staffed by eighty-five providers.

Management Directions of North Carolina (MDNC) is actively negotiating with other academic health centers in North Carolina to become a jointly owned venture that provides services on at least a statewide basis. MDNC currently manages 50 practices for 160 physicians, consults for 500 physicians, and manages 10 hospitals in 10 counties (figure 3). On-call nurse service is provided for ninety-seven providers in twenty-eight practices through a program called Registered Nurse Reassurance. This popular service decreases the need for physicians to answer after-hours calls by about 80 percent.

Leaders at Wake Forest believe it is very important to get primary care physicians to start thinking about how they would operate in a risk-taking capitated environment, which may develop in Winston-Salem, as well as in an essentially rural referral basin. Bringing about this change in thinking has proved to be difficult outside of the urban area, where there is as yet little or no managed care penetration.

QualChoice is a total risk-reward model for the physician and for the HMO. It is designed as shadow capitation. The total premium for each patient is assigned to a physician by a panel of from five to twenty physicians who must manage the entire premium even though the physician is providing service for what amounts to only 9–11 percent of the premium. Wake Forest's wholly owned medical center HMO is a for-profit entity, but it passes its profit on to the medical center in the form of dividends to a "holding company." This money is put back into its academic mission. This system allows Wake Forest to put HMO "arbitrage" back into the health care system rather than into "shareholders" in the for-profit sense, and also provides it with a "reality" site for the education of students and residents.

Medical center resources now involve a variety of subsidiaries, including home health care, home health subspecialists, home health solutions, radiographic imaging, and a nursing home. A geriatric facility was to be opened in February 1997. With this new center, the Sticht Center on Aging and Rehabilitation on the main campus, and an Outpatient Rehabilitation and Sports Medicine Unit within shuttle-bus reach, the medical center will have the vertical integration necessary to treat every level of care from cradle but not to the grave.

In terms of a horizontal structure, Wake Forest has the HMO, the practice network, the management services organization, and Regional Integrated Delivery System (RIDS), which is the holding company for these outreach activities. Wake Forest also maintains 75 specialty satellite outreach clinics in its service area in northwest North Carolina and southwestern Virginia.

In terms of physician services, the medical center created the Physician

Access Line five years ago. It is a toll-free number used by referring physicians to reach a specialist at the medical center. It guarantees that a caller can talk to a specialist in the discipline desired in less than five minutes. The university has received approximately 800,000 calls on that line. The service has also greatly contributed to increasing hospital admissions and appointments in the clinics of Wake Forest University Physicians. Perhaps more important over the longer term, approximately 60 percent of all calls have been for the purpose of receiving consultations, without charge, from our faculty specialists. Wake Forest leaders believe that the goodwill alone is worth the cost of the service.

Dual Strategy

Two independent, yet simultaneous, efforts are currently underway. The first is the development of a single or integrated clinical enterprise. This will require changes in the internal governance structure and will create an organization that aligns incentives within the medical center. An integrated enterprise will change the relationship of the physician and the hospital director with the trustees of the clinical enterprise, because a "parallelism" will be created with physicians and administrators as managerial partners appropriately throughout the system. All incentives for change and profit will be properly aligned to ensure that actions are predicated on the simple concept that we are in this together.

The second strategy is to establish new external alignments that will ensure the successful development of the RIDS. Administration and faculty leaders are currently exploring the need for alignments and identifying potential allies and partners. Wake Forest now has seventeen affiliated hospitals, plus a statewide partnership pending for MDNC.

The Regional Integrated Delivery System

The medical center is pursuing the RIDS strategy because it complements other major strategies that will enhance quality; deliver efficient, cost-effective care; and transfer leading-edge expertise (e.g., continuing medical education, telemedicine) to community clinicians. In addition, the system will create a network of health care providers that is attractive both to purchasers and to consumers of care. Therefore, the principal objective of RIDS is to increase the medical center's market share of patient care to accomplish the university's aca-

Figure 4.
RIDS MEDICAL CENTER RESOURCES, BOWMAN GRAY SCHOOL OF MEDICINE

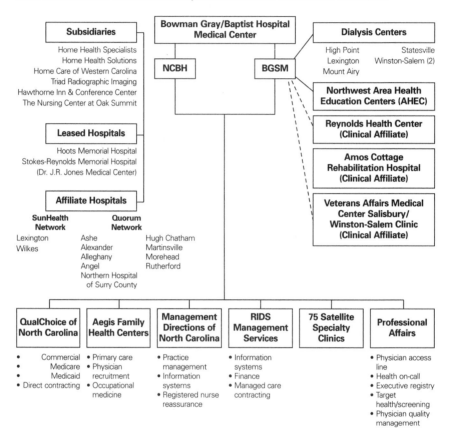

demic mission. Consequently, any RIDS initiative or investment must satisfy one of two criteria to be considered by medical center administrators: help secure additional covered lives for the enterprise or contribute to maintaining or enhancing the specialty referral systems.

Operationalizing RIDS will depend upon the degree to which the regional and internal strategies are successfully implemented. Figure 4 represents the outreach activities to be deployed. It will also require that the medical center establish an organizational unit to integrate RIDS within the medical center administrative structure to ensure integration of the practice plan (WFUP) with the hospitals and other service initiatives. This approach is depicted in figure 5.

RIDS is being developed according to regional design, thus recognizing local impact. The regional directors will live within the region they serve. The concept is similar to branch banking. It is an expensive proposition, and no medical center should attempt this approach unless it has sufficient capital that can be put at risk or a significant capital partner willing to share risk. For example, the regional information system (already in major pilot areas) has initial budget approval of $42 million.

KEYS TO SUCCESS

Many health care analysts and academic health center leaders have noted that academic health centers may need to dramatically change the manner in which they operate if the tripartite education, research, and service mission is to remain viable. The growth of managed care in academic health center markets

Figure 5.
PROPOSED ORGANIZATIONAL STRUCTURE OF THE REGIONAL INTEGRATED DELIVERY SYSTEM (RIDS).

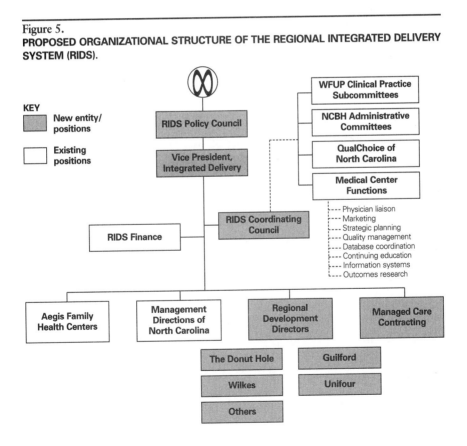

has forced tremendous changes in clinical service operations as well as the organization, governance, and financing of the research and education components of these institutions.

As noted by the University HealthSystem Consortium in its 1995 report, *Ownership, Governance, Organization, and Leadership of the Academic Health Center*, ultimate success and survival may depend on the degree to which these institutions are able to (1) take and manage financial risk, (2) build primary care capacity, (3) collaborate with other providers and insurers, and (4) demonstrate value to other organizations and the public in terms of cost, quality, and service. Success may also require that academic health centers build integrated delivery systems, thus increasing collaboration with other organizations. Finally, the expansion and use of information systems will be essential elements of success.

No single structural model will be perfectly adaptable to every academic health center and it is clear that academic health centers will have to link with multiple partners in new and different ways. Local political, economic, and social circumstances will determine the future direction for any individual institution because medical care in the United States is still a local issue.

A key factor in confronting change is the institution's governing board. Many experts have noted that most members of the board have to support rapid action, generally not a characteristic of people who hold trusteeship positions in not-for-profit institutions. Board members have to recognize that institutional leaders may make some mistakes and accept them as part of the decision-making environment. Inaction should be viewed as detrimental to the future of the institution. Strategic planning, as well as urgent planning, is needed to establish mechanisms that permit rapid decision making.

Leadership is the critical variable in managing such massive change. Leadership with a change-oriented style is needed. The most important characteristic in leadership is to be able to create a sense of readiness to change and an understanding of the need for change. Beyond the articulation of a vision, it is important to remember that change does not occur without acceptance by the people who are doing the work. The suits can't force change. Change can be made by only the white coats. We forget this at our peril.

CONCLUSION

This is an exciting time. People are going to have to learn the concept of shared autonomy. The next step for Wake Forest will be to increase the synergy within the academic health center in such a way that this massive clinical enterprise continues to support and enhance the academic mission. In a time of reduced clinical income and fierce competition for research funds, this will be no mean feat. Indeed, the will to change, although necessary, may not be sufficient: Legislation that recognizes the unique role of the academic health center in Wake Forest's health care system may be an eventual requirement. We must take every action to make sure that the backbone of modern American medicine does not, by neglect, get a bad case of osteoporosis.

Western University of Health Sciences

CREATING A NEW EDUCATIONAL ENVIRONMENT

ON AUGUST 9, 1996, THE COLLEGE OF Osteopathic Medicine of the Pacific (COMP) joined the College of Allied Health Professions and the College of Pharmacy to become Western University of Health Sciences (WesternU). A graduate nursing program was subsequently transformed into a college of nursing. The new university represents years of planning and is built on COMP's solid, primary care-oriented foundation. In the transformation to a university, COMP was seeking new advantages related to mission, function, culture, finance, and efficiency.

Three sections of this paper–Overview, Transition to WesternU, and New Designs for the Academic Enterprise–were written by Carl E. Trinca, PhD, professor of pharmacy education, vice provost/vice president for strategic planning at Western University of Health Sciences. Sage Bennet, PhD, associate professor of health professions, wrote New Designs for a Humanistic Educational Environment. The section on New Designs for a College of Pharmacy was written by Harry Rosenberg, PharmD, PhD, professor of pharmaceutical sciences and dean (chief facilitative officer); Patricia Chase, PhD, professor of pharmacy practice and facilitative officer for the Division of Professional Education; and Dr. Trinca. The final section, New Designs for Learning Anatomy, was written by Rafi Younoszai, PhD, professor of anatomy; Craig S. Kuehn, PhD, associate professor of anatomy, and Jonathan Leo, PhD, assistant professor of anatomy.

WesternU is a private, nonprofit institution. It has three campuses (Pomona, Chico, and Colton) and four colleges (osteopathic medicine, pharmacy, allied health, and nursing) that offer multiple programs and degrees. Sound financial planning and management, based on a tuition-driven model, have enabled the university to marshal the necessary resources to mount an impressive array of academic and community-based programs with only modest patient care revenues and philanthropic support. However, the university is currently pursuing an agenda of faculty and institutional entrepreneurship, including:

- a for-profit subsidiary in collaboration with the academic health center and a large physician management corporation;
- an alternative student loan program; and
- partnerships and strategic alliances with other colleges and universities and public schools for joint academic programs, collaborative scholarly endeavors, and shared resources (e.g., personnel, facilities, services, operations, purchasing).

COMP is one of 16 colleges of osteopathic medicine in the United States, and the only one in the West. The college was founded in 1977 on principles associated with the concept of "family," that is, small, close, respectful, caring, and nurturing. The establishment of COMP marked the successful culmination of efforts, begun in 1974, by the Society of Osteopathic Physicians and Surgeons of California "to seek the establishment of a College of Osteopathic Medicine in the state." The program was accredited by the American Osteopathic Association in February 1982, graduated its charter class of 36 students on June 13, 1982, and now enrolls more than 675 students.

In response to a growing demand for clinical educators, the college initiated a master of science in health professions education degree (MSHPE) program in 1986 and housed it within a newly created graduate division. The program promotes the knowledge and skills essential for competent teaching, as well as attitudes that foster continuing interest in education. Fourteen students, representing several health professions, are currently enrolled in the program.

The college accepted its first physician assistant (PA) class in February 1990. The graduate division became the Division of Allied Health Professions, and, subsequently, the School of Allied Health Professions. Current enrollment in the accredited, two-year primary care PA certificate program is 115 students.

COMP's School of Allied Health Professions enrolled 49 students in its charter physical therapy (MPT) program in January 1992. The twenty-eight-month program educates physical therapists to function as generalists concerned with wellness, health promotion, and humanism. The program is accredited and currently enrolls 158 students.

In 1991, COMP qualified as an academic health center because of its multifaceted programs in medical and allied health education and a newly forged relationship with the San Bernardino County Medical Center as its primary teaching hospital.

Beginning in 1988, the college elected to pursue regional accreditation by the Western Association of Schools and Colleges (WASC). The college is now accredited by the Accrediting Commission for Senior Colleges and Universities of WASC, an institutional accrediting body recognized by the Commission on Recognition of Postsecondary Accreditation by the U.S. Department of Education.

In January 1996, the college established its first regional campus in Chico, California, a community one hundred miles north of Sacramento. Among the issues considered during the planning for the establishment of a regional campus were the need for a rural program to complement the institution's largely urban-based program; the opportunity to innovate with various distance-learning technologies (computer-assisted instruction, the Internet, compressed video, and satellite); the need for advanced practice nurses in northern California; the need for accessible health professions educational programs in the region; and the desire to provide an educational program for family nurse practitioners. Two charter classes for physician assistants and master of sciences nursing/family nurse practitioner students each began their studies in Chico in January 1996. The certificate curriculum for physicians assistants is identical to the one offered on the Pomona campus and is delivered primarily via compressed video distance-learning technology. The nurse practitioner program is Internet based with intensive weekend classroom study on-site in Chico.

The College of Pharmacy enrolled its first doctor of pharmacy (PharmD) class in August 1996 with 65 students.

TRANSITION TO WESTERN UNIVERSITY

The transition to a university occurred against the backdrop of complex and changing health care and educational environments. The academic health center functioned in a system grounded in primary and community-based care, but with tremendous competing pressures from other providers. Efforts are now being directed at planning academic and service delivery programs in concert with the community, third-party payers, employers, and other health care providers.

The college had successfully focused its efforts and outcomes on teaching, while attaching less importance to research, community service, and entrepreneurship. Early in the transition process, however, it was acknowledged that the responsibilities of a university extend beyond excellence in teaching, and include the following prerogatives:

- Building high-quality, multidisciplinary health professions programs focused on teaching and learning; faculty-student interaction on a regular, ongoing basis; and the application of knowledge through practice and experience.
- Maintaining academic programs in the social context of ethos and good citizenship, caring, and humanism.
- Ensuring the discovery, application, integration, transfer, and dissemination of knowledge and technology in the basic and clinical sciences and health professions education.
- Fostering an environment for the detached, impartial evaluation of societal issues, particularly those surrounding health and disease.
- Ensuring a pool of specialized talent that the university makes available to government, industry, and the public.

The university structure also offers WesternU the opportunity to enhance efficiencies of operation. For example, shared student affairs functions, room scheduling, academic calendar maintenance, information services, integrated management information systems, and alumni affairs may offer economies of scale. Since it was conceived, the university has afforded students, faculty, staff, and administration of WesternU the opportunity to establish a new commonality of mission through greater shared responsibility. The university encourages greater collaboration among faculty, students, and administrators in the following areas: multidisciplinary teaching and scholarship; classroom, experiential, and service learning; and information resources and decision making. The institution is currently evaluating the formation of a single, university-wide faculty.

One teaching site has evolved into a hospital/clinic system, named the Center for Excellence in the Health Sciences, which has emerged as a centerpiece for the education and postgraduate training of health professionals. A separate corporation, with its own governance drawn from representatives of the medical center and university, has been created. Bylaws have been adopted and the resulting combined programs will offer the largest family practice residency program in the United States. A brand-new hospital will serve as the hub of a comprehensive, community-based health care delivery system beginning in 1998, and plans have begun to provide a presence for the university by construction of a clinical facility on the academic health center campus in Colton shortly thereafter. Other new academic endeavors, such as the two Chico-based programs, continue to provide the institution with valuable experience in the areas of collaboration and use of distance-learning methods.

Managing change seems to be the university's greatest challenge. Along these lines, certain infrastructure enhancements are in progress that will link campuses, enable better communication between academic units, and enable improved use of data and information. Most of these enhancements are resource-intensive and require balancing current needs against long-term comitments.

People, once thought to be a major source of institutional lethargy, seem willing to change as they are brought into the change process. Clearly, communications, opportunity for constructive input, and seeing the fruits of their labors are essential elements in involving students, faculty, staff, and administration. Not to be discounted is leading by example.

NEW DESIGNS FOR THE
ACADEMIC ENTERPRISE

Since the college of osteopathic medicine was founded, it has been dedicated to the preparation of health professionals qualified to provide comprehensive care to the family, to serve the primary care needs of the western United States, and to promote wellness, health, and community. At one time, the mission of the college to provide comprehensive family care was rare, if not unique, among health professions schools. Today, through self-awareness, public mandate, or market-driven forces, most academic health centers have adopted similar strategies, and WesternU is finding it more challenging to remain distinctive.

Transformation into the Western University of Health Sciences provided the necessary stimulus to examine such critical issues as mission, function, culture, finance, and efficiency in creative ways. In addition, the refocusing and reaffirming of the institution's humanistic mission, establishing a new College of Pharmacy, and exploring innovative learning methods have provided opportunities to redesign the educational environment. As a result, the restructuring and innovations described here can become a model for other institutions to follow and, thus, pave the way for the interdisciplinary and interprofessional education that will be required in academic health centers of the future.

The case discussions that follow describe the design of a humanistic educational environment, innovations in the design of a new pharmacy school, and a new approach for learning anatomy. Together, they provide examples of WesternU's attempts to take advantage of its environment, the transition to a university, and the willingness of individuals to commit to change.

NEW DESIGNS FOR A HUMANISTIC
EDUCATIONAL ENVIRONMENT

Three faculty members and the president of WesternU met in the fall of 1996 to discuss ways in which humanism could be more fully integrated into the campus community. Although a concerted effort toward humanism was new, a commitment to humanism already existed in the campus culture. This commitment was exemplified by the following attributes:

- high value placed on primary caregivers and their caring relationships with patients, colleagues, and students;
- a student-application process that identified students who were motivated to be compassionate and caring and evaluated nonscience majors as favorably as science majors;
- courses in medicine and literature, and ethics; and
- curriculum design for certain programs that integrated cross-cultural issues in medicine.

Building on the humanistic aspects that already existed in the campus culture, a more intensified focus began to emerge for integrating more fully into all aspects of campus life. Toward this end, several projects were begun, which in turn, generated other activities.

As the commitment to and enthusiasm about humanism began to grow, so did the circle of people who were discussing humanism with the president. What began with three faculty members soon included six, then the deans of the colleges, then an informal group of about ten to fifteen who went to dinner to discuss topics related to humanism. A working definition of humanism and answers to the question of "why humanism" began to emerge, as follows:

- Humanism is a way of caring that is fundamental to positive human interaction, and is manifested as a responsiveness to the needs of other human beings through respect, understanding, compassion, and empathy.

- Humanism is the foundation for excellence in the education of health professionals and a high quality of work life for administration, staff, faculty, and students.

- Working together in a humanistic environment provides the foundation for humanistic education.

- Humanistic education involves the cultivation of health professionals who can provide quality patient care that is respectful, compassionate, and empathetic.

- Staff, faculty, and administrators on campus need to model humanistic interpersonal relationships to experience a high quality of work life and to convey to students that humanism is valued.

- Creating an environment in which mutual respect and trust among all members of the campus community leads to open lines of communication and equitable treatment of people.

Formal vehicles were created to disseminate information and stimulate discussion about humanism on campus. Descriptions follow.

Journal of Humanism in the Health Sciences. The idea for the journal came out of informal discussions with the president. The goal is to provide a multidisciplinary forum for the presentation and exchange of ideas relative to humanistic, professional, and personal ethics, quality patient care, and health professions education. The journal's editor is a medical student who is assisted by a faculty advisor and an editorial board made up of faculty and students from the colleges of Western University. Articles are written and edited in a collaborative effort by students, faculty, and staff, and include research articles, essays, and poetry. The journal is published twice a year, in fall and spring, and discussions are underway to make the journal available on the Internet.

Humanism and Diversity Committee. This committee is made up of staff, faculty, and students from the colleges of the university. Guests from different parts of the campus and community are invited to committee meetings according to their interests. Participants exchange ideas about the meaning and scope of humanism and, from these discussions, several issues have been clarified, including the mission, goals, and special projects of the committee.

The commitee's mission is to serve as a focus for WesternU's learning about humanism and diversity by (1) defining, clarifying, and relating humanism and diversity in applied contexts; (2) translating the philosophy of humanism into action; and (3) devising, implementing, and evaluating projects that center on valuing the diversity and human-ness of the people on campus.

The committee goals are (1) to create a context for the exploration of issues that surround humanism and diversity; (2) to be a repository and clearinghouse for humanism and diversity issues, suggestions, and ideas; (3) to clarify and broaden the understanding of humanism and diversity on campus; and (4) to implement and communicate special projects and activities brought forth by members of the university.

Special committee projects now being considered include (a) discussion groups, colloquia, and scholarly research; (b) diversity etiquette guidelines; and (c) humanistic approaches to education and health care.

Library collection of articles on humanism. As interest in humanism grew on campus, a collection of articles from staff, faculty, and students was started. A notebook of articles on humanism was created for campuswide reading. Copies of the articles are also disseminated to members of the humanism and diversity committee for reflection and discussion.

Distinguished Lecture Series on Humanism. Dr. Andrew Weil, author of the best-selling book, *Spontaneous Healing,* was the first speaker in the lecture series. There was an excellent attendance of over 450 faculty, students, and staff and great potential for discussion and exchange of ideas. Recommendations for speakers in the distinguished lecture series and for other contexts on campus are going through the committee for review.

Assessment projects. A natural outgrowth of the humanism-on-campus activities are assessment projects. Three projects are underway.

1. In an outcomes project, Assessing Humanism, a consultant is studying available instruments for assessing humanism and selecting the most appropriate and valid method of determining the effect of humanistic education on WesternU graduates.

2. A student in the Master of Science in Health Professions Education program is preparing a survey to study humanistic attitudes of osteopathic physicians and the role that education plays in the development of humanistic caregivers.

3. Assessment tools are being researched to determine the effects of producing humanistic physician assistants through the integration of cross-cultural issues in medicine in the curriculum.

By integrating humanism into the university culture, providing humanistic education to health professionals, and actively implementing projects that enhance humanism, WesternU distinguishes itself as a twenty-first century leader in innovative health professions education.

NEW DESIGNS FOR A COLLEGE OF PHARMACY

When academic planning began for a new pharmacy program in 1991, the profession was experiencing extraordinary tension between education, accreditation, and large employers, notably chain drug stores. These tensions focused on the level of professional preparation (BS versus PharmD), workforce supply and future demand (including pharmacy technicians), scope of practice (dispensing versus pharmaceutical care), and technology. Every indication was for continuing strong demand for pharmacists practicing in both traditional and evolving roles.

In addition, managed care has had a serious impact on the profession. As a result, it has been suggested that traditional pharmacy roles may not be sustainable at their current level. For example, utilization rates for pharmacists in managed care organizations tend to be significantly lower than in other settings, and technology may offer efficiencies and economies that could change the current workforce requirements. Finally, an oversupply of pharmacists may develop in the health care system.

According to anecdotal evidence, some students who graduated in 1995–96 did so without the benefit of multiple job offers. These professional and market issues gave added incentive to developing innovative plans for the pharmacy program.

Traditional teaching methods and curricula were reviewed in designing the new program. The lecture format, in which professors talk and students listen, has serious shortcomings when the needed competencies and the ability to provide pharmaceutical care are considered.

The importance of such competencies and abilities as critical thinking, problem solving, decision-making, communicating effectively, self-learning, and locating and using information mean that student- and learning-oriented curricula and teaching methodologies should be used. Such a design suggests that the faculty must

- encourage and guide students to use the rich   information resources available;
- maximize essential faculty-student interaction through the use of active learning formats;
- integrate new technologies fully into the student learning process; and
- enhance student collaborative or peer learning.

At the Western University of Health Sciences College of Pharmacy such restructuring of the traditional faculty-oriented role was accompanied by a number of fundamental changes described below.

Organizational and Administrative Structure

The College of Pharmacy is organized into three functional divisions: Professional Education, Professional Practice, and Graduate Education and Scholarship (figure 1). Participatory leadership for each division is provided by its facilitative officer who reports to the chief facilitative officer. Together, the facilitative officers comprise the leadership team of the college and meet formally as the Executive Committee.

Functionally, the facilitative officer for the Division of Professional

Figure 1.
ORGANIZATIONAL STRUCTURE, COLLEGE OF PHARMACY, WESTERNU

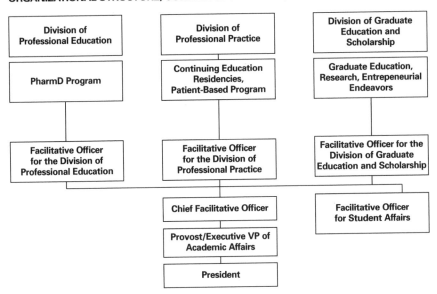

Education has oversight responsibility for all educational aspects in the PharmD program, and the facilitative officer for Graduate Education and Scholarship has responsibility for all matters related to scholarship, including research and graduate education, and entrepreneurial activities. The facilitative officer for the Division of Professional Practice provides the leadership for activities associated with experiential programs, continuing pharmaceutical education, and residencies. Facilitative officers are participatory leaders who involve, support, and empower others, build consensus, and get commitment from those they lead. They act as facilitators, helping the faculty solve problems and make decisions.

Faculty are not assigned to a particular division. Rather, their association with a division is dependent on the activities of that division. For example, a faculty member's instructional endeavors in the PharmD program fall under the purview of the Division of Professional Education; his or her participation in the patient-based program falls under the purview of the Division of Professional Practice; and his or her involvement in research activities falls under the purview of the Division of Graduate Education and Scholarship.

The organizational structure for the college is intended to

- flatten the hierarchy, thereby streamlining the decision-making process;

- eliminate overlapping responsibilities, thereby minimizing organizational conflict; and

- empower the faculty, thereby enhancing the potential for collaboration, creativity, and entrepreneurism.

Curriculum Design and Delivery

The curriculum is organized into a number of broad-based components (figure 2).

Core academic program. This is the central educational component of the first three years of the PharmD curriculum. It represents an integrated approach to pharmaceutical education taught by teams of clinical and basic science faculty and provides fundamental biomedical and pharmaceutical principles as well as a knowledge base of disease and pharmacotherapy. It consists of five core academic programs, A-E, representing major content areas that, in turn, are further divided into subject areas.

Figure 2.
PHARMD CURRICULUM, COLLEGE OF PHARMACY, WESTERNU

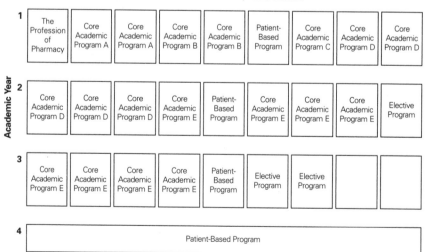

A. Biochemistry and Molecular Biology
- Enzyme Structure and Function and Structural Proteins
- Bioenergetics and Membranes
- Mitochondrial Oxidative Metabolism
- Carbohydrate Metabolism
- Lipid Metabolism
- Nitrogen Metabolism

Molecular Biology
- DNA Replication
- RNA Synthesis
- Protein Synthesis
- Regulation of Gene Expression
- Gene Transfer

B. Biological Basis of Disease
- General Pathology
- Immunology
- Mechanisms of Infection

C. Metabolism and Nutrition

D. Fundamentals of Therapeutic Agents
- Receptor Theory
- Pharmacodynamics of Major Drug Classes
- Pharmaceutics
- Biopharmaceutics
- Pharmacokinetics

E. Management of Homeostasis
- Nervous System
- Cardiovascular
- Pulmonary
- Renal

- Gastrointestinal
- Endocrine/Reproductive
- Hematology
- Infectious/Neoplastic Diseases
- Rheumatology

The Pharmacist Development Program is a longitudinal, problem-based learning component of the PharmD curriculum that is designed to introduce students to the complex nature of the emerging health care system. This program is intended to assist students in developing abilities that will be critical in enabling them, as future health care practitioners, to respond both to patients and their environments. Students focus on the following subject areas:

- Health Care Economics and Finance
- Health Care Systems/Managed Care
- Total Quality Management
- Outcomes Measurement
- Biostatistics
- Epidemiology and Population Health
- Ethics and Jurisprudence
- Clinical Policy Analysis
- Wellness, Health Promotion, and Disease Prevention
- Medical and Drug Literature Evaluation/Informatics
- Interpersonal Skills and Concepts of Human Behavior

The elective program (area of concentration) component allows students the opportunity to pursue in-depth areas of concentrated study.

The patient-based program begins with early student involvement with patients and builds toward intensive clinical practice experiences in the clerkships of the final year. The emphasis in this program is the development of the clinical skills necessary for the provision of pharmaceutical care. The following subject areas are included:

- Interviewing and Counseling Skills
- Physical Assessment
- Problem Solving and Decision Making
- Computer Use in Clinical Practice
- Continuity of Care

- Advisor/Advocate Program
- Pharmacy Practice Experiences

Allocation of Academic Time

As shown in figure 2, the PharmD curriculum is delivered in the block form. The academic year is divided into nine 3 1/2-week blocks with a four- to five-day break between blocks. Each day students are engaged in active learning formats with faculty and peers for six hours.

The block system offers several advantages:

- It provides students the opportunity to read, hear, discuss, reflect, and study intensely without distraction from other subjects.
- The amount of class time each day (6 hours) offers opportunity for, and demands, varied class activities, especially active modes of learning, with time for discussions, case presentations, simulations, role playing, debates, group projects, and other activities that encourage active participation. Such activities foster student interest and motivation.
- It is conducive to the development of interpersonal skills because students are encouraged to work together several hours a day.

Evaluation and Assessment

Assessment is multifaceted, including both traditional and nontraditional methods to monitor effectiveness in achieving the curricular goals established for the PharmD program. It is centered on students achieving higher levels of competencies than are required in most other pharmacy programs.

On the traditional level, standard quizzes and examinations, primarily essay-type, are administered. Additionally, students are evaluated on written reports, poster presentations, and oral presentations. Students maintain a personal portfolio with examples of their best work. The portfolio is reviewed with the student by their faculty advisor on a quarterly basis.

Nontraditional methods include evaluation, remediation, and collaborative activities. Student evaluations are completed on a quarterly basis with data describing progress obtained from peer (team) evaluations, self-evaluations, and review of grades. The faculty mentor assigned to each student meets and discusses progress, and develops a performance plan for the student's continued progress. Portfolios are also reviewed at this time.

The College of Pharmacy has established very high standards for its students. Each student must achieve a minimum of 90 percent on all exams, quizzes, and papers and as a final block grade. Failure to meet this standard requires remediation. In remediation, the student meets with the faculty member responsible for the assignment and is required to demonstrate the ability to successfully answer questions similar to those missed on an examination. Papers must be rewritten until 90 percent is earned. This intermediate intervention ensures that students keep pace with their classmates and do not fall behind in their studies.

The curriculum is student-centered and each student is assigned a team. Teams of five to seven students collaborate to complete assignments such as case projects, posters, and presentations. Students are responsible for teaching other teams and class members. To encourage collaboration, there are several block assignments, both social and academic, that require teams to work together.

Design of the Physical Environment

The design of the facility contributes greatly to the establishment of the desired student-centered environment. The College of Pharmacy has been allocated 60,000 square feet of space in the Health Professions Center, which is currently being remodeled. Classrooms dedicated to the PharmD program are configured as either a hexagon or a pentagon with seats facing inward, away from walls. This design allows students to see each other and creates an inclusive atmosphere that encourages interaction and discussion among students. Moreover, instructors can move around freely, see each student clearly, and talk with them directly.

Multimedia equipment with projection capabilities occupy the central area of each classroom. Projection screens are suspended from the ceilings. Located on the perimeter of each classroom are several break-out rooms, which are assigned to teams of students for small-group discussion, peer teaching, and self-directed study. The classrooms and break-out rooms will have access to Internet and other on-line electronic databases. Each student is equipped with a notebook computer.

NEW DESIGNS FOR LEARNING ANATOMY

Gross anatomy instruction in medical school has traditionally held a dominant position in the curriculum. However, the usual curriculum of 200–300 hours of factual and lecture-intensive coursework has recently been challenged. First, geometric increases in biomedical knowledge has forced a compensative reduction in anatomy contact credit hours. Second, the need to prepare generalist physicians with new competencies has required even anatomists to explore teaching methods that take advantage of active self-learning, problem-solving, critical thinking, and greater communication skills.

The American Association of Clinical Anatomists (AACA) was formed in 1984, in part, to respond to these challenges. Its position paper* and several recent innovative programs serve as important examples of trends in anatomy instruction. Generally, there has been a shift away from relying heavily on memorization toward problem-solving, from principally passive to more active learning, and toward teaching future physicians how to communicate. Further, the AACA and the Basic Science Educational Forum (BSEF) have strongly recommended that medical schools make anatomy clinically oriented in order for students to see the relevance of anatomic detail in their future medical practices.

The Human Gross Anatomy course at WesternU's COMP has been taught in a traditional format to ensure that its students, as future osteopathic physicians, gain a thorough knowledge of anatomy. With its compacted first-year curriculum, one of the challenges faced by the anatomy faculty is to maintain high standards in anatomy and, at the same time, to increase student morale, reduce stress, and promote self-learning and critical thinking in a small-group discussion format.

The gross anatomy laboratory, where four students are assigned to each table, provides the ideal setting to observe and assess these goals. Currently, many students come into the anatomy laboratory without adequate preparation and rely on the faculty to perform dissections and explain to them what they have to learn, while students just watch. This situation is not conducive to active learning, and also deprives the other twenty-eight students assigned to the faculty member of equal attention; clearly, something needs to be done to encourage students to actively dissect and learn about anatomy hands-on, and it must be done with the faculty available.

---

*Bears, O.H.; R.A. Chase; and R.Ger. 1986. Gross Anatomy in Medical Education. *American Surgery* 52: 227-332.

Additionally, the gross anatomy laboratory lends itself to topographic and surface anatomy instruction whereby students can locate, palpate, and auscultate internal organs while, at the same time, studying them within the body through dissection. In this manner, students learn to use anatomical landmarks for physical examination well before they begin their clinical rotations.

It is for these reasons that we have designed and implemented two new approaches for teaching and learning anatomy.

Surface Anatomy Curriculum

Ideally, when a physician examines a patient, he or she should have something akin to x-ray vision: the ability to see where bone, muscle, and organs are, or at least should be, located in the patient. Obviously, this is not possible in a literal sense, and even real x rays give only a limited anatomical view. But the physician must, nonetheless, know where everything *should* be located. Too often, students are presented with static images, no surface landmarks, and body parts distorted through embalming or prior removal. Since osteopathic physicians rely on the patient's anatomy to make a correct diagnosis, knowing precisely where bone, muscle, and organs are located is a critical part of a student's learning. Therefore, it is important to take time during regularly scheduled gross anatomy laboratory to study surface anatomy and properly emphasize the value of this method in gathering patient information.

Because using anatomic landmarks to assist in diagnosis is so important to osteopathic physicians, instructional goals have been established for first-year students. First, locate and palpate surface landmarks for important internal structures, including bony prominences, muscles and tendons, and internal organs; and second, use clinical case studies to show students how anatomical information relates directly to their medical practice, and to teach proper charting procedures and basic skills of physical diagnosis such as palpation, auscultation, and percussion. This method makes anatomy more interesting and relevant to the student's clinical interest.

Five different body regions (upper limb, thorax, abdomen, pelvis and perineum, and head and neck) are covered in twelve one-hour sessions. During each session, a case study is presented in a standard SOAP format, reinforcing proper charting procedures and the use of clinical terminology. Students then learn how to palpate, percuss, and auscultate the area under study, using each other as models and for practice. Lastly, the students learn to prescribe both traditional and osteopathic treatments, whichever is indicated.

Intensive Summer Anatomy Course

Demonstrated competence in gross anatomy is absolutely essential to continuing in medical school and, often, students must be remediated or tutored if they are to be able to continue their studies. WesternU has used two methods to retain its students: a basic summer anatomy program, designed for students without prior human anatomy coursework to bring them up to speed before the regular course begins each August; and a tutorial program that involves second-year medical students assisting first-year students. The basic summer anatomy program has proven useful, but its benefits are limited by enrollment capacity; time constraints on second-year medical students lessen the usefulness of the tutorial program.

A third method, an intensive summer anatomy course, is being implemented. This program targets a select group of students for instruction prior to the school year, thus creating a group of advanced students who guide and encourage fellow first-year students in the regular anatomy class. The course has two goals. First, those students who take the course will receive more exposure and, therefore, presumably a much better understanding of anatomy, both by repetition and because they have to assist their fellow students in understanding the material. The second goal is to encourage those students who perform well during the summer intensive course to serve as facilitators for the rest of the students in the first-year class. As such, they help lessen anxiety as well as improve the overall knowledge of the first-year student population. It should be noted that the student facilitators are not truly teachers per se, but are there also to learn through interaction with other students; further, student facilitators do not serve as replacements for faculty or alter student-faculty ratios. The result should be greater summer student understanding through increased exposure, and greater first-year student understanding through more efficient interaction with both faculty and summer students.

Course planning is complete, and forty students were to matriculate in June 1997, commencing seven weeks of intensive instruction on human anatomy. The course includes two hours of lecture and three hours of laboratory daily, Monday through Friday. Four days a week there will be one hour of discussion on the clinical correlation of anatomic structure. The course will earn students 10.5 semester credits, of which an additional four credits (for a normal course total of 14.5), will be earned by working with the first-year medical students in the fall. Four examinations will be given: back, shoulder and upper limb; thorax and abdomen; pelvis and lower limb; and head and neck.

The final four credit hours will be awarded based on specific criteria. For example, students earning a grade of A or B must attend lectures and labs; in the labs they serve as facilitators and perform two prosections. Their responsibilities include initiating discussion and guiding students to correct solutions; they do not participate in dissection because it is a learning activity in which they have already participated. They perform prosections on hard-to-dissect structures such as the perineum or the parasympathetic ganglia of the head. Prosections are only demonstrated to other students after faculty review. Performance is assessed on completeness, and the grade for these four credits is averaged with the grade for the summer anatomy course in determining the final course grade. Students earning a grade of C during the summer course are required to take all laboratory exams with the regular students to determine the final course grade. Students receiving a D, or unsatisfactory, grade will have to take the entire, regular human gross anatomy course and their grade will be determined by their performance in the course.

The summer program offers such benefits as greater time to study other subjects during the regular term and experience in teaching others. Also, students will receive scholarship support to defray the expenses associated with tuition and course fees.

Benefits also accrue to other students. For example, students failing the regular human gross anatomy course can remediate through the summer intensive course and continue their second-year of medical school with their entering class. For our Osteopathic Manipulative Medicine Fellows, the summer course can serve as a refresher course. And, lastly, all students completing the summer course can assist with anatomy-related research.

As WesternU gains experience with the summer-intensive anatomy course, fine-tuning will occur. The main criterion for determining future direction is what is best for the student.

The Medical College of Wisconsin

REPOSITIONING A PRIVATE, FREESTANDING ACADEMIC HEALTH CENTER FOR THE 21ST CENTURY

T HE MEDICAL COLLEGE OF WISCONSIN (MCW) IS A private, freestanding academic health center in Milwaukee affiliated with twenty-seven hospitals and other health care institutions throughout the state. The institution does not own a hospital, but has four major affiliated hospitals. They are Froedtert Memorial Lutheran Hospital (MCW's primary adult, acute care hospital); the Veteran's Administration Medical Center (in Wood, Wisconsin); the Children's Hospital of Wisconsin (the only tertiary pediatric hospital in the state); and the Milwaukee County Mental Health Complex (a 1,000-bed psychiatric hospital that is the largest hospital in the state). In 1996, Milwaukee County closed John L. Doyne county hospital, one of MCW's major affiliates. Doyne Hospital facilities were purchased by Froedtert.

MCW is only one of two academic health centers in a state with a population of approximately five million people. The other is the University of

---

This report is based on a presentation by T. Michael Bolger, JD, president and CEO of the Medical College of Wisconsin, at the 1996 symposium on The Future of Academic Health Centers of the Association of Academic Health Centers in Chicago.

Figure 1.
TOTAL BUDGETED REVENUES, MCW, INC., 1996–97

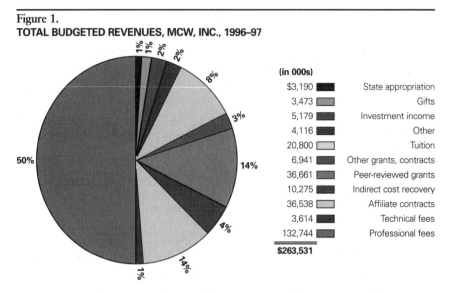

(in 000s)		
$3,190	■	State appropriation
3,473	▨	Gifts
5,179	■	Investment income
4,116	■	Other
20,800	▢	Tuition
6,941	■	Other grants, contracts
36,661	▨	Peer-reviewed grants
10,275	■	Indirect cost recovery
36,538	▢	Affiliate contracts
3,614	■	Technical fees
132,744	▨	Professional fees
$263,531		

Wisconsin-Madison Center for Health Sciences, a public institution. MCW is in a standard metropolitan statistical area of about two million people in southeastern Wisconsin. It has a full-time faculty of about 850, a volunteer faculty of about 1,200, and 3,000 employees. It is the anchor for the Milwaukee Regional Medical Center, which has 12,000 employees and a combined $1 billion annual budget.

MCW has its roots in two proprietary medical schools: the Wisconsin College of Physicians and Surgeons and the Milwaukee Medical College, both of which were established in the late 1800s. The Wisconsin College of Physicians and Surgeons, the first school to enroll medical students and grant valid degrees in the state of Wisconsin, opened in May 1893 with a faculty of twenty-two. The Milwaukee Medical College opened in September 1894 with a faculty of twenty and an enrollment of ninety-six. Both institutions were members of the Association of American Medical Colleges. Following the recommendation of the Council on Medical Education of the American Medical Association, the two medical schools merged in 1913 to become the Marquette University School of Medicine, with an enrollment of 270 students. Marquette University graduated its first class from the School of Medicine in 1913, awarding seventy-eight MD degrees.

In September 1967, it became apparent to Marquette University that state funds were needed for the survival of its medical school, but the state was unwilling to use its funds to support a private, religious institution. Therefore, the Marquette board of directors created MCW as an independent, freestanding medical school. In 1978, the college moved from the Marquette University campus to the campus of the Milwaukee Regional Medical Center. In late 1991, the board of trustees of MCW approved a proposal to coalesce the college's graduate programs into a graduate school, later named The Graduate School of Biomedical Sciences. The graduate school currently grants the PhD degree, as well as the MS, MA, and MPH degrees. It has a full-time dean who reports directly to the president of the college.

THE BUDGET

The revenues of the MCW budget totalled approximately $263 million in 1996-97 (figure 1). Revenues include state appropriation of approximately $3 million, which supports family medicine; gifts of about $3 million; and investment income of about $5 million. Other income, including gifts and money from patents, of about $4 million; tuition income of about $20 million and grants and contracts of approximately $7 million; peer-reviewed grants of $36 million; indirect cost recovery of about $10 million; technical fees of about $3 million; and professional fees or clinical income of approximately $132 million, that account for about 50 percent of the total budget, highlighting the institution's disproportionate dependency on clinical income.

Revenues from affiliate contracts with MCW's hospital partners amount to approximately $36 million. Affiliate contracts are primarily associated with clinical revenue growth because the hospitals pay MCW for services rendered. The revenue from the affiliate hospitals consists of $17.5 million annually from Froedtert, $8 million from Children's Hospital, and about $11 million from the

Figure 2.
AFFILIATE BUDGETED REVENUE, MCW, INC., 1996–97

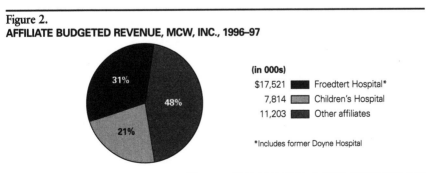

(in 000s)

$17,521 ■ Froedtert Hospital*
7,814 ▨ Children's Hospital
11,203 ■ Other affiliates

*Includes former Doyne Hospital

Figure 3.
TOTAL BUDGETED EXPENSES, MCW, INC., 1996–97

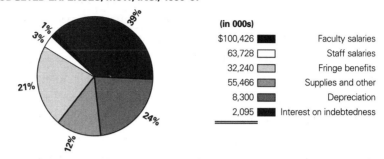

(in 000s)		
$100,426	■	Faculty salaries
63,728	☐	Staff salaries
32,240	▦	Fringe benefits
55,466	▨	Supplies and other
8,300	■	Depreciation
2,095	■	Interest on indebtedness

other affiliates (figure 2). The affiliated hospitals are squeezing those numbers as hard as they can. The money is used to pay program directors, faculty salaries, department chairpersons, and administrative staff for the hospitals. Very little of the affiliate contract money goes to support research and academic activities. MCW has an academic enrichment fund, called the dean's tax, which in 1996–97 equalled 11 percent of fundable revenues. From the faculty viewpoint, this is a large sum.

Total budget expenditures for 1996–97 were about $262 million, of which 39 percent went for faculty salaries, 24 percent for staff salaries, 12 percent for fringe benefits, 21 percent for supplies and other items including research, 3 percent depreciation, and 1 percent for interest on indebtedness (figure 3). Close to two-thirds is related to salaries.

MANAGED CARE

One of the biggest concerns for MCW is the impact of managed care. The growth of managed care is slowly eroding MCW's referral base (figure 4), with Wisconsin rapidly catching up to Minnesota in terms of managed care penetration. The Duluth Regional Health Care System has been gaining an increasing share of the market in northwestern Wisconsin. The Marshfield Clinic has penetrated north-central Wisconsin, Wausau Hospital System is moving rapidly into the northeastern sector, and the Mayo Clinic and Gundersen Clinic is each seeking a market share in the southwestern part of the state. Physicians Plus and the Dean Clinic, both headquartered in Madison, are trying to extend their markets, which have the potential to hurt the University of Wisconsin. Eastern Wisconsin is what MCW would normally consider its catchment area. The Aurora Health

System, a large multidisciplinary integrated delivery system, is emerging in the areas near Kenosha and Racine, and has resulted in some new hospital alliances. This balkanization of the state by health care providers has shut out academic medicine, which is perceived as being expensive and unfriendly to patients. Thus, MCW has found itself in a tug-of-war with other health providers that should be allies.

THE STRATEGIC PLAN

MCW recently completed a strategic plan that will require $100 million in new monies to fund. Another $15 million will be needed from the affiliated hospitals. Essentially, the new strategy is to increase primary care capacity, reduce costs, attack expenses, develop advanced information systems, participate in integrated delivery systems, and prepare to accept as much risk as possible. MCW also needs to provide access to a full range of health care services in a variety of delivery settings.

The risk issue is a key to the future. Academic health centers are allergic to risk, and it is very important for these institutions to begin to develop their risk-taking abilities.

Academic health centers also have not demonstrated cost-effective patient care management very well. Part of the reason for MCW's shortcomings in that area was the lack of a unified clinical practice. Five years ago, MCW established a unified clinical practice at the medical school. However, the new practice group still operates in the old medical fashion, with departments holding a great deal of power, thus making effective functioning difficult.

The academic health cen-

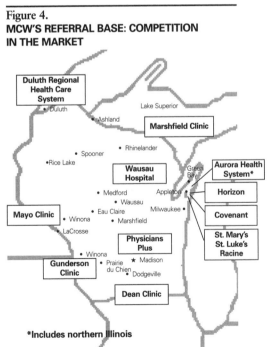

Figure 4.
MCW'S REFERRAL BASE: COMPETITION IN THE MARKET

*Includes northern Illinois

ter's biggest challenge is to maintain the education, research, and service missions in the wake of a highly competitive and market-driven environment. As part of its strategic plan, MCW, in partnership with Froedtert and Children's Hospitals, is developing primary care sites around metropolitan Milwaukee and southeastern Wisconsin for teaching, research, and clinical service purposes. This development is one way of rebuilding referral sources, as it has required increased outreach and work with the community and community physicians at the new sites. The distribution of these sites is a key element in future success.

Currently, Froedtert Hospital is a closed-staff hospital. All staff members must be faculty members of the MCW medical school. This also holds true for Children's Hospital for all subspecialties, and the Veteran's Administration Medical Center for all departments. Froedtert Hospital, with support from MCW, recently created a community practice division within its medical staff. All community-based specialists must be accredited, but they will not necessarily have to be appointed to the faculty, at least not to the full-time faculty.

MCW also needs a competitive cost structure. Froedtert Hospital is currently the highest-priced hospital in Wisconsin in terms of delivery of care, and the MCW faculty also tend to deliver expensive care in outpatient settings. Froedtert Hospital is very concerned about education and societal costs. Societal costs include indigent care, which is approximately 6 percent. According to Froedtert, the hospital contributes 12 percent of its $306 million budget to the Medical College of Wisconsin for educational and research purposes. Froedtert's contributions to MCW largely cover the cost of supervising residents, but also include the administrative duties that MCW faculty assume at the hospital. These costs put the hospital at a significant disadvantage with respect to other hospitals and systems in the community.

Academic health centers need to increase the volume of clinical services, if they are to survive. However, in the rush to increase clinical volumes and revenue streams from clinical income, academic health centers sometimes forget that the reason for such activity is not just to make money, but to preserve their mission.

Health care delivery is moving away from inpatient care and toward ambulatory care. Inpatient facilities are becoming highly specialized with high technology medicine that requires significant capital investment to continue to compete for a shrinking pool of patients. Academic health centers will need access to capital to build such facilities.

MCW's access to capital is diminished because it does not own a hospital. When hospitals were making money, many were able to save a war chest that could be used to buy primary care practices or enhance a primary care network. MCW does not have that option, but it does have ways of affiliating itself with primary care institutions that do not want to be engulfed by a large, integrated delivery system.

As one of only two academic health centers in the state, MCW has to use its monopoly power wisely to ensure that it is a value-added component for other integrated delivery systems. That concept is starting to take hold. The Aurora Health Care System and the Covenant Health Care System, neither of which is affiliated with MCW, have approached MCW about the possibility of joint programs. Such talks are not only the result of self-interest but also community interest.

MCW leaders believe that academic medicine must survive if medicine is to survive. There is also some enlightened thinking about developing a community pool of funds from all the integrated delivery systems to help academic medicine survive in ways that are good for the community. Although these concepts have not been put into writing, there are some signs that these large integrated systems understand the value that academic health centers bring to the marketplace.

Academic health centers deliver excellent health care services, but do not always deliver the hotel services that many patients use as a measure of quality, such as prompt scheduling and good manners. MCW is looking at these aspects of its service, which needs improvement. In terms of costs, the clinical practice plan recognized that cutting expenses was not sufficient if MCW were to be competitive. Thus, MCW is developing advanced information systems that are essential for the future; MCW leadership is convinced that you cannot manage what you cannot measure.

MCW leaders have also worked very hard to develop strong community ties. One advantage to being a private institution is not having to answer to a State Board of Regents, which is often the case with public institutions. MCW has a board of trustees comprising thirty-one people. While it has taken ten years to build this board, it has been well worth the time and effort. The board members are among the most powerful people in Milwaukee and the state. For example, the board includes the president and CEO of Northwestern Mutual Life, the president and CEO of Johnson Controls, and the president and CEO of Wisconsin Energy. It is a real asset to have that kind of power on the side of the academic health center and its leaders. These people have influence that can be very important and helpful in dealing with other organizations and enterprises in the state. The board is critical to the success of MCW.

MARKET STRATEGIES

MCW's current market strategies include enhancing its decision-making processes. Cumbersome decision-making structures are a major problem for academic health centers today. It is crucial for these institutions to have leaders with decision-making authority and to have structures in place that permit rapid decision making. If academic health center leaders are not empowered, they are not going to be able to function effectively in rapidly changing markets.

MCW is seeking to expand its educational opportunities and provide more venues for education and training of its students. It is also scrutinizing its academic programs in terms of size, quality, and stability. For example, MCW and its affiliated hospitals are currently addressing the size of their residency programs. Cuts in the neighborhood of 10–20 percent are anticipated over the next several years. MCW currently has about 750 residents; with cuts over the next two years, there will be about 600 residency positions at the school. These decreases in residents will require a concomitant cutback in faculty, which leads to the question of where to cut faculty. The institution is wrestling with the issue. It believes that most of that cutback can come from natural attrition, rather than a wholesale reduction in force. MCW is also revisiting the issue of class size. It currently enrolls 200 medical students every year, but perhaps should reduce this number to approximately 170; no decision has been made yet.

CONCLUSION

The two watchwords for the future are agility and balance. Academic health centers have to be agile in the marketplace even as they try to create balance within their systems. Academic health centers cannot and should not give away their expertise in specialty and subspecialty medicine because it is this expertise that distinguishes them and that, ultimately, adds value to them and to any systems of which they are a part.

Appendix B

1997–1998
AHC QUESTIONNAIRE

Association of Academic Health Centers
STUDY OF THE ORGANIZATION, GOVERNANCE, AND STRUCTURE OF ACADEMIC HEALTH CENTERS, 1997–1998

We are requesting that the AHC member respond to the survey. Please do not pass this instrument on to your staff.

I. Institutional Leadership/Management

1. Do you have direct line authority over (i.e., the authority to hire or fire) the dean/director of:
   - ☐ school of allied health
   - ☐ school of dentistry
   - ☐ school of medicine
   - ☐ school of nursing
   - ☐ school of pharmacy
   - ☐ school of public health
   - ☐ graduate studies
   - ☐ hospital administrator
   - ☐ others: (*please list*) _____
   _____

2. Do you have the power to hire/fire the directors of any of the following:
   - ☐ development/fundraising
   - ☐ finance
   - ☐ government relations
   - ☐ human resources

☐ marketing
☐ planning
☐ public relations/public information

3. Which of the positions in #2 do you share with the university? *(please list)*

_____ _____

_____ _____

_____ _____

4. Do you have access to flexible funds which allow you to initiate new programs and stimulate change in your institution? ☐ Yes ☐ No
   If yes, what is the approximate annual amount: $ _____

5. Do you have the power of the budget? ☐ Yes ☐ No
   If yes, can you shift funds from one health professions school to another? ☐ Yes ☐ No

6. a. Does the academic health center have single-signature contracting capability to commit the academic health center's clinical enterprise (including hospital) to managed care contracts? ☐ Yes ☐ No

   b. Who has the signature authority? *(title)* _____

7. What are your primary mechanisms for capital formation (e.g. bonding authority, gifts, loans)? _____

   _____

8. In the last two years, have there been any changes in your capacity to form capital? ☐ Yes ☐ No
   If so, what _____

9. Is your institution allowed to acquire debt? ☐ Yes ☐ No
   If yes, what level of authorization do you have for acquiring debt?

   _____

   _____

10. Do you have adequate capital to meet your education, research, and service goals?　□ Yes　□ No

11. How have service contracts (e.g., security, maintenance) with your parent university or university system changed within the last year?
□ Increased　　□ Stayed the same　　□ Decreased
This change represents a $ _____ loss/gain (circle one) to the academic health center.

II. Governance

12. Please list governing boards within the university, academic health center (including primary teaching hospital and practice plan), and health network/system on which you sit.
Please X boards for which you are the chair, XX boards on which you can appoint members, and XXX boards where you have authority to designate the chair

_____ 　　 _____

_____ 　　 _____

_____ 　　 _____

13. Is the board of directors/trustees/regents that governs the academic health center: (*check all that apply*)
□ Elected? by whom? _____
□ Appointed? by whom? _____
□ Self-perpetuating?

14. a. Is the academic health center governed by: (*check one*)
□ university or university system board of trustees/regents
□ own governing board
□ other

b. *If governed by the full university board, does the academic health center have:*

☐ an advisory board comprising university trustees with power to recommend budget/policies but no governing authority

☐ a subset of the board with governing authority

15. Does the academic health center have:

a health system or network governing board?　　　☐ Yes　☐ No

a visiting committee of external and/or
community advisors?　　　☐ Yes　☐ No

16. In the past year, have governance structures of the academic health center changed? ☐ Yes　☐ No
If yes, how? (please explain):

_____

_____

17. In the past year, have hospital and/or clinical services governance structures changed?　　☐ Yes　☐ No
If yes, how? (please explain):

_____

_____

III. Health Professions Education

18. What percentage of *funding for education* comes from the sources listed below?

School	State Funds (%)	Tuition (%)	Clinical Revenues (%)	Other (%)
Medicine	%	%	%	%
Allied Health				
Dentistry				
Nursing				
Public Health				
Pharmacy				
Other				

19. Has state funding for your educational programs in the past year:
    ☐ Increased   ☐ Stayed the same   ☐ Decreased
    a. If *increased*, by what amounts: _____% $ _____
    b. If *decreased*, by what amounts: _____% $ _____

20. How has the level of your primary teaching hospital's support of the educational programs changed over the *past year*?
    ☐ Increased   ☐ Stayed the same   ☐ Decreased

21. How is basic science education organized in your academic health center?
    ☐ each health professions school has its own departments
    ☐ medical school faculty teach students from other schools/programs
    ☐ academic health center-wide (students from various professions learn together)
    ☐ university-wide
    ☐ other (*specify*) _____
    _____

22. Other than basic sciences, are there shared courses across the health professions schools/programs?   ☐ Yes   ☐ No
    If so, what? _____
    _____

23. a. In the past year have you *downsized* any of the following in your medical school and residency programs? (*check if yes and all that apply*)
    ☐ FT faculty
    ☐ class size
    ☐ specialty residency programs
    ☐ fellowship programs

    b. Have you *downsized* any of the following in your other schools and programs? (*check if yes and all that apply*)
    ☐ FT faculty (which schools) _____
    ☐ class size (which schools) _____

    c. Have you closed any schools or programs in the past year?
    ☐ Yes   ☐ No
    If yes, which ones?

    _____
    _____

24. Have you *expanded* any of the following in the past year (*check if yes and all that apply*)
    ☐ nursing programs (*which ones*) _____
    ☐ physician assistant program _____
    ☐ other schools/training programs (*please list*) _____
    ☐ teaching sites in the community _____
    ☐ other (*please explain*) _____

25. Does the academic health center have enough ambulatory sites for education of:
    medical students?   ☐ Yes ☐ No
    other health professions students?   ☐ Yes ☐ No

26. Have you made any changes in the tenure system in the past year?
    ☐ Yes   ☐ No
    If so, what _____

27. Do you have post-tenure reviews? ☐ Yes ☐ No
    If yes, were they mandated by the state legislature? ☐ Yes ☐ No

28. Have you changed the basis for the compensation system in the past
    year?
    For Faculty? ☐ Yes ☐ No
    For Staff? ☐ Yes ☐ No
    If so, how _____

    _____

    _____

29. In the past year, has there been any change in the reward system to fos-
    ter the following activities?
    (*check if yes and all that apply*)
    ☐ education/teaching   ☐ community-based activities
    ☐ multiprofessional activities ☐ basic research
    ☐ health promotion/disease prevention ☐ clinical research
    ☐ primary care   ☐ health services research

IV. Research

30. Is your research enterprise self-sufficient? ☐ Yes ☐ No
    If no, what amount needs to be subsidized from other sources?
    _____ % $ _____   ☐ Not sure

31. Have you established new alliances, joint ventures, or partnerships in the
    past year to support the research enterprise? (does not relate to grants or
    short-term relationships) ☐ Yes ☐ No
    If yes, what? _____

    _____

    _____

    b. Anticipated level of support _____

32. Have you established or disbanded any centers of excellence in the last two years?

☐ Established (*which ones*) _____

☐ Disbanded (*which ones*) _____

33. How are decisions made regarding the *allocation of financial support and capital equipment* for research? (*check if yes and all that apply*)

☐ on an academic health centerwide basis

☐ by school

☐ by department

☐ other_____

_____

34. How are decisions made regarding the *allocation of research space?* (*check if yes and all that apply*)

☐ on an academic health centerwide basis

☐ by school

☐ by department

☐ other _____

_____

35. Do you have a technology transfer office?   ☐ Yes   ☐ No

36. Do you have a policy giving researchers financial incentives to engage in entrepreneurial activities?   ☐ Yes   ☐ No

37. What was the approximate amount of royalties paid to the academic health center last year?

$ _____   ☐ Not sure

38. How are royalties distributed?

Percent (%) to: ☐ investigator _____% other(s): _____%

☐ department _____%   _____%

☐ school   _____%   _____%

V. *Clinical Services*

39. Do you have a single comprehensive, multispecialty group practice?
    □ Yes   □ No
    If no, are you working to develop such a practice?
    □ actively implementing   □ in the conceptual stage
    □ not doing anything yet
    If yes;
    Does your practice plan have a:
    single patient record   □ Yes   □ No
    single billing and collection system   □ Yes   □ No
    single appointment system   □ Yes   □ No

    Is the practice plan billing and collection system integrated with hospital billing and collection?   □ Yes   □ No

    Are health professionals other than physicians involved in the practice plan or plans?   □ Yes   □ No
    If yes, which professions _____
    _____

    Is there single governance structure for the practice plan?
    □ Yes   □ No

    Is there a single governance structure for the hospital and the practice plan?   □ Yes   □ No

    To whom does the head of the practice plan report? (**give title**)
    _____
    _____

    What is the composition of the governing body of the practice plan? (**list by title**)
    Chair _____   _____
    _____   _____
    _____   _____

40. The following populations represent what percentage of admissions to your primary teaching hospital?

Medicare _____%   ☐ Not sure

Medicaid _____%   ☐ Not sure

Uninsured _____ %   ☐ Not sure

41. What was the amount of uncompensated care provided in your primary teaching hospital last year?

$ _____   ☐ Not sure

42. How high is the managed care penetration in your academic health center's service area?

☐ 0–10%   ☐ 41–60%

☐ 11–25%   ☐ 60%+

☐ 26–40%   ☐ Not sure

43. What percentage of admissions to your primary teaching hospital last year were patients in a capitated program? _____%   ☐ Not sure

44. Does the university own its primary teaching hospital? ☐ Yes ☐ No

    If less than 100% ownership, please explain _____

    _____

45. Has the status/ownership of your primary teaching hospital changed in the last year?   ☐ Yes ☐ No

    If yes, check which of the following applies:

    ☐ merged with a nonprofit hospital

    ☐ merged with or acquired by a nonprofit health system

    ☐ merged with a for-profit hospital

    ☐ merged with or acquired by a for-profit health system or hospital chain

    ☐ formed a new entity with a nonprofit hospital to control clinical service management

    ☐ became a state or public authority

    ☐ other _____

    _____

46. In the past year, have you *downsized* any of the following in your primary teaching hospital?

    (check if yes and all that apply)

    ☐ number of active beds

    ☐ number of licensed beds

    ☐ nursing staff

    ☐ other staff

47. Do you currently have a university-owned HMO?　☐ Yes　☐ No

    a. *If yes, when was it established?* _____

    b. *Is your HMO a:* ☐ *staff model* ☐ *PPO* ☐ *other*

    c. *If no, did you have an HMO in the past?* ☐ Yes　☐ No

    d. *If you had one, when was it sold?* _____

48. Do you currently have an institution-owned insurance product?

    ☐ Yes　　☐ No

    a. *If yes, is it wholly owned / partially owned?* (**circle one**)

    b. *If no, do you plan to develop one in the next year?* ☐ Yes　☐ No

49. What linkages do you have with the following health care providers? *(please check all that apply)*

PROVIDERS	LINKAGES					
	Bought	**Merged with**	**Formed partnership with**	**Affiliated with**	**Contracted with**	**Held discussions with**
Other hospitals						
Community-based physicians						
Community health centers						
Entities that bring substantial number of covered lives						
Academic health centers in the same city, state, or region						

50. Are you part of a network or health system? (i.e., an interrelated or inter-

connected group of providers, including hospitals, physicians, and other clinical sites that have contractual agreements to deliver specific services) *(check one)*

☐ Yes, for all clinical services

☐ Yes, for some clinical services/product lines *(please list)*

_____

_____

☐ No, not part of a network/system

51. Do contractual agreements with new clinical partners provide support for any of the following?

    (check if yes and all that apply)

    ☐ medical education

    ☐ graduate medical education

    ☐ other health professions education

    ☐ indigent care

    ☐ research

    ☐ other (explain) _____

    _____

Name: _____

Institution: _____

CONFIDENTIALITY

Please note that all information will be pooled for purposes of analysis so that individual institutions will not be identified or identifiable, unless you grant permission to cite examples from your institution. Please indicate your prefer-ence: ☐ OK to cite   ☐ Do not cite

Please return by fax or mail to the AHC **no later than July 3, 1997.**

    Attention: Serena Curry
                    Manager of Information Technology
                    Association of Academic Health Centers
                    1400 Sixteenth Street, NW, Suite 720
                    Washington, DC 20036
                    Telephone: (202) 265-9600 Fax: (202) 265-7514